Treating
Chronic
Pain

Pill-Free Approaches To
Move People From Hurt To Hope

CBT – Mindfulness – Essential Treatment Tools
Worksheets – Exercises - Assessments

Martha Teater, MA, LMFT, LPC, LCAS • **Don Teater**, MD, MPH

Copyright © 2017 by Martha Teater and Don Teater

Published by
PESI Publishing & Media
PESI, Inc
3839 White Ave
Eau Claire, WI 54703

Cover Design: Amy Rubenzer
Layout Design: Amy Rubenzer & Bookmasters
Edited By: Blair Davis

Printed in the United States of America

ISBN: 9781683730927

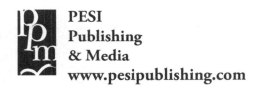

PESI
Publishing
& Media
www.pesipublishing.com

Dedication

With much love to Nora

... and those who may come after

Acknowledgements

We gratefully acknowledge the encouragement, support, and suggestions of many people who have influenced us in the writing of this book. For his pioneering work in the treatment of chronic pain and his professional generosity, kudos go to Dr. John Otis. For early cheerleading, we salute Dr. Trent Codd and Dr. John Ludgate from the Cognitive-Behavioral Therapy Center of Western North Carolina. For her stalwart friendship and keen insights into the world of publishing, a round of applause goes to Dawn Cusick of Dawn Cusick Books. For her patient and wise guidance throughout the entire process from proposal to publication, we give a hearty shout-out to Karsyn Morse of PESI Publishing.

We would know nothing of value about treating chronic pain if not for the inspiration we've gained from working with those in pain. For allowing us a front-row seat to witness their healing and recovery, we rise to give a standing ovation to the many people we've worked with as they've moved from hurt to hope.

And, most importantly, we thank our family. We are blessed by your unfailing love and unconditional support. You are the brightest light and greatest joy in our lives. It's with overwhelming gratitude that we thank you for all you mean to us. Thank you, Kevin, Luke, Betsey, Nora…and those who may come after.

Martha Teater
Don Teater

Table of Contents

. . . .

About the Authors

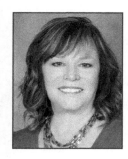

Martha Teater, MA, LMFT, LPC, LCAS, is a licensed marriage and family therapist, a licensed clinical addictions specialist, and a licensed professional counselor. She has been in private practice in western North Carolina since 1990, most of those years in a primary care setting. Martha has worked in outpatient substance abuse and mental health, with a free clinic, and with medication-assisted treatment.

Martha has provided hundreds of trainings across the United States and internationally on the behavioral treatment of chronic pain, evidence-based treatment of trauma, the *Diagnostic and Statistical Manual of Mental Disorders*, 5th edition, compassion fatigue, and other topics.

An active Red Cross volunteer, Martha serves in both disaster mental health and Service to the Armed Forces supporting military families.

A prolific writer, Martha has published more than 175 articles in newspapers and magazines, including *Psychotherapy Networker* and *Family Therapy Magazine*. She is coauthor of *Overcoming Compassion Fatigue: A Practical Resilience Workbook* (PESI, 2014).

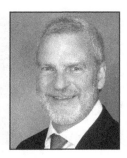

Don Teater, MD, MPH, is a family physician who has lived and worked in western North Carolina since 1988. Don and Martha have worked together in a fully integrated practice for the majority of their professional careers. Don initially practiced the full range of family medicine but has gradually migrated to working entirely with people who have addiction and mental health disorders. He is a national expert in the areas of pain, addiction, and opioids. He has worked for the past five years with the Centers for Disease Control, the National Safety Council, and many other state and federal agencies and community organizations on the opioid issue.

In June 2016, Don founded Teater Health Solutions to concentrate on educating prescribers and others on the science of opioids and how that should influence treatment and policy decisions. He continues to work one day per week treating those afflicted by the disease of addiction at Meridian Behavioral Health Services in Waynesville, North Carolina.

Preface

As a behavioral health professional, you've probably worked with many people who have chronic pain. Estimates are that about a third of Americans experience this, so it's likely that they've sat with you in your office. Without specialized training, you may feel out of your element as you try to intervene. Your frustration may mount as you see limited progress or questionable motivation. You may wonder about your own abilities and scramble to offer tools that might help.

When your client is on opioids, your challenges are compounded. How do you know if your client is using them appropriately? Are opioids the best medications for their pain? How can you encourage your client to reduce their reliance on pain pills when they say that they are the only thing that helps?

As a therapist I've experienced the challenges of helping people with chronic pain improve their lives. I've also felt a boost in confidence as I've sought out training and education to enhance my skills. Having powerful tools leads to much more robust outcomes for the people we work with.

This book offers you solid, evidence-based approaches that work. As you see the changes that result, you will feel much more capable, effective, and optimistic. As an added bonus, you'll know that you are helping people make dramatic changes in their lives.

— Martha Teater

I have been treating pain as a family physician since I started seeing patients in 1988. I know of several individuals that ultimately died from the opioids that I started them on for their pain. The scary thing is, I had no idea what I was doing when I was treating their pain or giving them opioids. Even though the most common reason people go to the doctor is for pain, we receive almost no education in treating pain in medical school or residency.

For the past five years, I have been working on the issues of chronic pain and opioids and have been speaking to and educating prescribers. Everything that I am teaching them is information that I did not know for the first 25 years of my practice. It is all new to most of them as well.

My key point to prescribers is that medications are not very good for treating pain. Especially with chronic pain, medications have very little use. Behavioral therapy is key. Therapists can reduce pain more than any doctor can. I tell these prescribers that it is imperative that they urge their patients with chronic pain to see a behaviorist who is trained in the treatment of pain; without behavioral interventions, there is little hope that the person will get better. Their response to me is always, "We don't know who to send them to who's trained in pain treatment."

This book is a result of those conversations. Currently, the default treatment (and also the most harmful and least effective) for chronic pain is opioids. By changing this norm to behavioral therapy, we will not only treat pain better, we will save lives.

— Don Teater

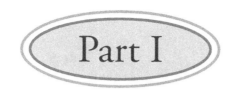

Part I

Introduction to Treating Chronic Pain

The combination of pain, opioids, and addiction is the triune scourge of the United States in the 21st century. In our society today, all three of these problems are closely related, and we cannot address just one without paying attention to all three.

This problem began in the 1990s, when the medical community started prescribing more opioids in an honest attempt to better treat pain. A major challenge is that physicians get very little training and have very little understanding of pain, opioids, or addiction. Since the onset of increased prescribing, we have had more pain, more opioid use, and more addiction than ever before. The "cure" has become the problem.

Science shows us that the answer to these issues lies within the behavioral health community. Pain is a complex biopsychosocial disease. Healthcare in the United States is heavily focused on treating the physical aspect of disease, but it does not do well at integrating the psychosocial aspect. By treating the psychosocial component of pain, we can reduce the pain AND the suffering more effectively than with any medication. The guidance provided by this book can revolutionize your care of people in pain.

This book is geared toward supporting behavioral health professionals working with people who have chronic pain. We want to emphasize that there are many people who live well in spite of having chronic pain. As you look at how they are able to do that, you'll probably notice that they are already doing many of the things that we suggest in this book. These individuals are probably socially connected, active, engaged, and avoiding the use of pain pills. While we focus on clinicians, this book is also useful for people with chronic pain, as it offers multiple worksheets that can be completed alone or with a professional.

The goal of this book is to help therapists become the cornerstone of pain treatment. Pain treatment should be multimodal, but individuals suffering from pain must learn that the solution lies within themselves with guidance from the behavioral community and consultation from the medical community.

By using this approach, we can reduce pain, addiction, and the number of opioids prescribed. When we impact that triune scourge, we will know that we are truly making a difference for individuals, families, and communities.

Understanding Pain

> *"True compassion means not only feeling another's pain but also being moved to help relieve it."*
> —*Daniel Goleman*

America has a pain problem. Pain surrounds us. Most of us know someone with chronic pain. That should not be surprising. Pain is a part of the human experience; it always has been. How each person *reacts* to pain may be different and is largely based on community, religious, and ethnic norms.

Pain is an unpleasant feeling that is experienced by everyone at various times in life. In the United States, pain is a significant health problem. The Institute of Medicine estimates that more than 100 million Americans report frequent or chronic pain. Economic costs from pain alone are estimated to be between $560 and $635 billion each year. Pain is the most common reason for people to seek medical care.

So, what is pain, really? Surprisingly, pain is more difficult to define than you may think. Because everyone has experienced pain, we all have some idea what it is; however, because our experiences are different, our ideas of pain are also different. According to the International Association of the Study of Pain (IASP), pain is *"An unpleasant sensory and emotional experience associated with actual or potential tissue damage, or described in terms of such damage"* (IASP Taxonomy, 2017). Notice that pain has both sensory and emotional aspects. There are also cognitive (thinking) and memory components. It is extremely important to understand that our interpretation of our own pain is so much more than just the sensory aspect, which we can rate on a 0-to-10 scale. Our emotions, thoughts, and memories all have a profound impact on how we are *affected* by the physical pain we experience. They also contribute to how much pain we *actually feel*.

ACUTE VERSUS CHRONIC PAIN

As we try to understand pain, it is critically important to realize that acute pain is completely different from chronic pain. **Acute pain** is a normal physiologic response to tissue damage or potential damage. An example of potential damage would be if your hand comes too close to the burner on the stove and you feel the pain from the heat but pull your hand away fast enough that no damage occurs. Acute pain serves a purpose—it protects us from tissue damage and helps us attend to areas that are injured so they may heal. As our bodies heal, the acute pain goes away—the pain has served its purpose.

Chronic pain is completely different. It is not normal and does not serve a function. Chronic pain continues after healing has occurred and does not serve as protection any longer. Often, the exact cause of chronic pain is unclear. Chronic pain usually leads to behavior that is not helpful. The person with chronic back pain tends to be less active and tries to avoid further pain, when in fact increased activity is more beneficial in decreasing the pain. Chronic pain is not helpful. It just hurts.

ACUTE PAIN

- From tissue damage
- Resolves as tissue heals
- Lasts less than 3 months

CHRONIC PAIN

- Etiology often uncertain
- Continues even though tissue has healed
- Lasts more than 3 months

HOW DO WE FEEL PAIN?

Nociceptors are the first step in our sensing of pain. The word *nociceptor* comes from the Latin word *nocere*, which means "to harm." Nociceptors are nerves that sense harm or a threat of damage to our tissues. When activated, they carry a signal all the way to the spinal cord. For some areas of our body—such as our toes—the nerve cell may be several feet long. These are the nerves that are damaged in diabetes, resulting in dysfunction that can result in either pain (if they are overactive) or numbness (if they do not work at all).

The nociceptors travel all the way to the spinal cord, where they activate the second nerve in the pathway, the **spinothalamic nerve**. It is called *spinothalamic* because it carries the nerve impulse from where the nociceptor has entered the spine to an area in the middle of the brain called the *thalamus*. The purpose of this nerve is only to transmit the signal from the nociceptor to the brain—it is a relay. Spinothalamic nerves are those that are affected when you receive spinal or epidural anesthesia. The anesthetic blocks these nerves at the area where it is administered so all nerve signals that began below that level are interrupted, resulting in numbness below the area of the block.

The spinothalamic nerves carry the signal to the **thalamus**. The thalamus is like a 911 center for a community; it receives the signal then transmits it to the necessary areas of the brain to allow for an appropriate response to the threat. The thalamus sends the signals to many areas of the brain, but the ones on which we are focusing are the somatosensory cortex (physical pain), the limbic system (emotions), the frontal cortex (thoughts), the hippocampus (memory), and the amygdala (fear).

The nerves that go from the thalamus to the somatosensory cortex are the **somatosensory nerves** (SS nerves); these are *the most important* nerves in the process of feeling pain. Activation of these nerves is what causes us to feel the physical sensation of pain. *This is critically important to understanding pain.* If the nociceptor is activated but there is some interruption of the signal before it reaches the brain (as with regional anesthesia or a spinal cord injury), we will not feel any pain. On the other hand, if the nociceptors are not activated but the SS nerves are activated by another source, we will experience pain just as though there is actual tissue damage! This is important to understand because in many cases of chronic pain, the nociceptors are NOT activated, but an abnormal process has caused the SS nerves to fire, resulting in the very real sensation of pain. The SS nerves are the "bad guys" in chronic pain. ***In this book, we focus on efforts to prevent the activation of the SS nerves and reduce their impact when they do activate.***

The image shown here depicts how the sensory cortex in the brain is laid out. If a brain surgeon were to touch the area of the brain where we sense pain in our elbow, this would activate the SS nerves and we would feel pain in our elbow—even if there is nothing wrong with our elbow.

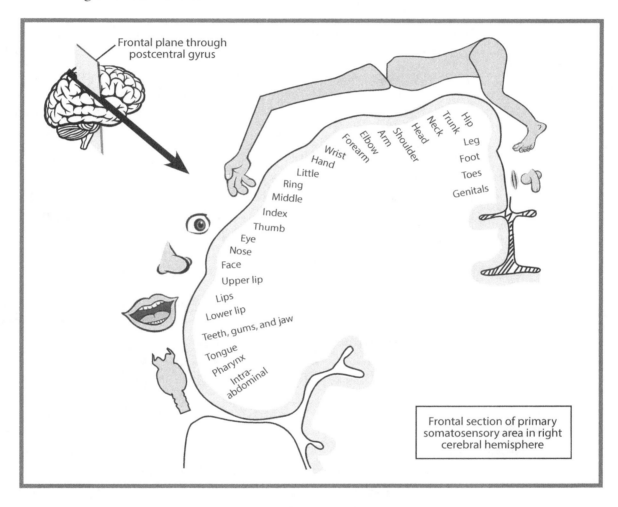

Nerves from the thalamus also go to many other areas of the brain, including the amygdala, frontal cortex, limbic system, and hippocampus. These areas are all important in helping us deal with pain and avoid further pain. There are multiple complex connections between these areas that either augment or decrease the intensity of pain. However, in chronic pain, these connections become problematic. The SS nerves become easily activated by nerves coming from these other areas of the brain. By controlling our thoughts and emotions, we can decrease signals to our SS nerves and actually experience less pain. This explains why behavioral therapy is so important in managing chronic pain.

Acute Pain

Acute pain almost always follows the appropriate pathway. The nociceptor nerve is activated by some type of tissue damage or potential damage. The nociceptor nerve sends a signal to and activates the spinothalamic nerve, which then sends a signal to the thalamus, activating the SS nerves and causing us to feel pain. We then take whatever action is needed to relieve the pain and protect our tissues. This is the way that pain is supposed to work!

Chronic Pain

There are three major causes of chronic pain, and each is determined by which portion of the pain pathway is problematic:

- **Nociceptive pain.** The pain is coming from continued stimulation of the nociceptive receptor.
- **Neuropathic pain.** The pain is coming from problems with the nerve transmission from the nociceptor to the thalamus. This may be from damage to either the nociceptor (as with diabetic neuropathy) or the spinothalamic nerves (as with a herniated disk).
- **Central sensitization pain (CSP).** This is the most common and the most problematic cause of chronic pain. The somatosensory nerves in the brain become extra sensitive and fire when they should not. This results in real pain even though the problem does not originate where we feel the pain. For example, if the somatosensory nerves located in the region of the brain that feels pain in the neck become abnormally activated, real pain is felt in the neck: It is not imagined but does not originate from actual damage in the neck.

Chronic nociceptive pain is usually caused by ongoing inflammation but is usually not debilitating. It may be seen with chronic arthritis of the joints. This pain can usually be controlled with anti-inflammatory drugs (such as ibuprofen) and acetaminophen. When this pain is debilitating, there is almost always coexisting CSP.

> The somatosensory nerves in the brain become extra sensitive and fire when they should not. This results in real pain even though the problem does not originate where we feel the pain.

Chronic neuropathic pain is caused by damage to the nerve between the tissue and the brain. This damage causes irritation to the nerve and causes it to fire excessively, resulting in pain. If the nerve is damaged to the point where it does not function at all, numbness occurs. Neuropathic pain may be controlled with drugs that stabilize nerve tissue, such as the antiseizure medications gabapentin and carbamazepine. Chronic neuropathic pain can be severe but usually is associated with some CSP.

Central sensitization pain is completely different. CSP does not occur because nerves are damaged but because they have *changed*. The somatosensory nerves and the nerves that activate them have been altered by some outside factor. We don't know everything that can cause this but suspect that childhood trauma, adult trauma, prolonged exposure to opioids, and prolonged exposure to pain are some of the triggers. Because of their increased sensitivity, these nerves may be activated when they should not be. The thalamus becomes like a supercharger, taking minimal input and releasing maximal output. This can lead to several problems:

1. **Increased activation.** The positive and negative feedback systems malfunction, causing increased signals to the SS nerves. Even light touch that activates just a few of the nociceptors is greatly magnified and activates many SS nerves, making the light touch feel like severe pain. When I (DT) used to examine patients with low back pain and press lightly on their lumbosacral muscles, I would often see them wince or cry out in pain. I thought they were purposely magnifying their response in an effort to get opioids prescribed. Now I realize that most of these people were experiencing central sensitization, and my light touch was truly magnified by the neurons in their brain to feel like I had hit them with a baseball bat. I apologize to these former patients for my disbelief. Unfortunately, few medical providers understand CSP, and most continue to respond as I did.

2. **Inappropriate activation with no input from the proprioceptors.** The SS nerves receive input from spinothalamic nerves but also from many additional nerves, including those that come from the limbic system (emotions), the frontal cortex (thinking and decision-making), the hippocampus (memory), and the amygdala (memory and fear). With central sensitization, the SS nerves may be activated without *any* input from spinothalamic nerves but instead from the other areas of the brain. When this happens, stress, anxiety, depression, worry, bad memories, or other events can cause pain that feels exactly the same as if there were damage or trauma to the tissues. After all, these are activating SS nerves. For example, someone with CSP may experience severe back pain that is not originating in the back. Instead, it is coming from the stress they are experiencing at work. It is important that our clients understand that this pain is real and not imagined. A recent study found that when physicians destroyed the nociceptor nerves causing low back pain by using radiofrequency ablation, there was no reduction in pain (Juch et al., 2017). That is because most people with chronic low back pain have a significant component of central sensitization.

We now know that ongoing pain actually changes the brain. We call these **neuroplastic changes**. The brain does not grow new nerve cells after we are born, but it does change connections between neurons and increase or decrease nerve pathways. These changes lead to many of the characteristics of CSP, in which our emotions and thoughts have more impact on activation of the somatosensory nerve than do the nociceptors.

Adverse childhood experiences (ACEs) may also lead to many neuroplastic changes during childhood. This explains why people with higher ACE scores have more pain as adults.

Of the various types of *chronic* pain, CSP is by far the most significant. It is the major component in chronic back pain, chronic daily headaches, whiplash, and fibromyalgia. It is probably a factor to some degree in all types of chronic pain. With

> Think of central sensitization like the volume control of an electronic device set on "high." No matter the input, the output will be very loud. By reducing the volume control in central sensitization, we can reduce the pain output.

CSP, it is very clear that people are not imagining their pain. When medical providers recommend that someone see a counselor or psychologist, the individual may think that the provider believes it is "all in their head." This is not the case. The pain is real, but it is being stimulated or enhanced by parts of the brain other than those related to tissue damage in the area from which the pain is felt. Thus, it can be reduced by decreasing the input from the emotional, cognitive, and fear centers in the brain.

Almost all chronic pain involves a combination of two types of pain. CSP is likely a factor to some degree in all chronic pain. There may also be a component of nociceptive pain or neuropathic pain. Chronic arthritis is nociceptive pain that is originating in the inflamed joints but is made worse by CSP. The amount of CSP varies from individual to individual and may be the primary driver of the amount of pain people feel. For chronic low back pain, CSP is likely the greatest source of the pain. If we are treating someone whose chronic low back pain is primarily caused by CSP with epidural injections and surgery, the outcome on pain will not be significant. In fact, studies have shown that epidural steroid injections are no better than placebo for the treatment of chronic back pain.

PAIN TYPES AND PROGNOSIS		
Type	**Example**	**Prognosis**
ACUTE		
Nociceptive	Ankle sprain	Good
Nociceptive + CSP	Minor injury but severe pain	Guarded—may develop chronic pain
CHRONIC		
Nociceptive	Osteoarthritis—non-limiting	Usually mild chronic pain
Nociceptive + CSP	Osteoarthritis—limited activity	Chronic pain leading to "sick role"
Neuropathic	Herniated disc—leg pain, tolerable	Surgery may help
Neuropathic + CSP	Herniated disc—back pain, intolerable	Poor—surgery likely to fail
CSP predominant	Fibromyalgia or chronic back pain	Poor without multidisciplinary treatment

Even pain *after* cancer treatment can be largely from CSP. People diagnosed with invasive cancer are frequently prescribed opioids for the treatment of pain. Two thirds of these patients survive the cancer, and many remain on opioids for "post-cancer pain." After pain treatment, there is often little reason for people to continue to have pain. A significant component to ongoing pain is likely CSP. This is such a significant problem after cancer treatment that some researchers have developed an inventory to evaluate CSP in patients with post-cancer pain (Nijs et al., 2016).

Case Example

Jason – A Cautionary Tale

I (DT) once had a patient who had been injured in a traffic accident. This had resulted in severe trauma to his foot. He had immediate surgery and was in a cast and a wheelchair for six weeks. Jason's pain continued during that time and was managed with opioid pain medications. Following removal of the cast, activity was gradually increased, but pain prevented him from bearing full weight on his ankle. He continued on crutches—and opioids. He also had been diagnosed (prior to his accident) with chronic anxiety and depression. Jason saw a mental health professional for this and a podiatrist for his ankle.

Over the course of the next 10 years, he had eight more operations on his foot and ankle. None relieved the pain. Finally, the podiatrist did an amputation below the knee. Can you guess how he did following surgery? His pain continued. His chronic pain had changed his brain. He now had a large component of central sensitization and was probably also having opioid withdrawal pain during attempts to reduce the amount of medication he was taking. If fewer opioids and more behavioral therapy had been used early in his treatment, his outcome likely would have been much better.

THE CENTRAL SENSITIZATION INVENTORY (CSI)

How can you determine how much CSP is contributing to someone's pain? **The Central Sensitization Inventory (CSI)** may be used to determine severity of CSP. The CSI consists of 25 questions and may be self-administered. Each question may be answered as follows: Never (0 points), Rarely (1 point), Sometimes (2 points), Often (3 points), or Always (4 points). Total points reflect the severity of the CSP. Following is a breakdown of score ranges and the intensity of CSP they represent.

Subclinical:	0 to 29
Mild:	30 to 39
Moderate:	40 to 49
Severe:	50 to 59
Extreme:	60 to 100

The CSI has two parts, Part A and Part B. For scoring purposes you will only look at the 25 questions in Part A. Part B was initially used to help correlate the results with previous diagnoses. For our purposes it adds additional clinical background information but isn't included when the instrument is scored.

CSI Inventory (Part A)

Name _____   Date _____

Please circle the best response to the right of each statement.

	Never	Rarely	Sometimes	Often	Always
1. I feel tired and unrefreshed when I wake from sleeping.	Never	Rarely	Sometimes	Often	Always
2. My muscles feel stiff and achy.	Never	Rarely	Sometimes	Often	Always
3. I have anxiety attacks.	Never	Rarely	Sometimes	Often	Always
4. I grind or clench my teeth.	Never	Rarely	Sometimes	Often	Always
5. I have problems with diarrhea and/or constipation.	Never	Rarely	Sometimes	Often	Always
6. I need help in performing my daily activities.	Never	Rarely	Sometimes	Often	Always
7. I am sensitive to bright lights.	Never	Rarely	Sometimes	Often	Always
8. I get tired very easily when I am physically active.	Never	Rarely	Sometimes	Often	Always
9. I feel pain all over my body.	Never	Rarely	Sometimes	Often	Always
10. I have headaches.	Never	Rarely	Sometimes	Often	Always
11. I feel discomfort in my bladder and/ or burning when I urinate.	Never	Rarely	Sometimes	Often	Always
12. I do not sleep well.	Never	Rarely	Sometimes	Often	Always
13. I have difficulty concentrating.	Never	Rarely	Sometimes	Often	Always
14. I have skin problems such as dryness, itchiness, or rashes.	Never	Rarely	Sometimes	Often	Always
15. Stress makes my physical symptoms get worse.	Never	Rarely	Sometimes	Often	Always
16. I feel sad or depressed.	Never	Rarely	Sometimes	Often	Always
17. I have low energy.	Never	Rarely	Sometimes	Often	Always
18. I have muscle tension in my neck and shoulders.	Never	Rarely	Sometimes	Often	Always
19. I have pain in my jaw.	Never	Rarely	Sometimes	Often	Always
20. Certain smells, such as perfumes, make me feel dizzy and nauseated.	Never	Rarely	Sometimes	Often	Always
21. I have to urinate frequently.	Never	Rarely	Sometimes	Often	Always
22. My legs feel uncomfortable and restless when I am trying to go to sleep at night.	Never	Rarely	Sometimes	Often	Always
23. I have difficulty remembering things.	Never	Rarely	Sometimes	Often	Always
24. I suffered trauma as a child.	Never	Rarely	Sometimes	Often	Always
25. I have pain in my pelvic area.	Never	Rarely	Sometimes	Often	Always
Total Each Column					

Overall Total [   ]

CSI Inventory (Part B)

Name _____   Date _____

Have you been diagnosed by a doctor with any of the following disorders?

Please check the box to the right for each diagnosis and write the year of the diagnosis.

		No	Yes	Year Diagnosed
1	Restless Leg Syndrome			
2	Chronic Fatigue Syndrome			
3	Fibromyalgia			
4	Temporomandibular Joint Disorder			
5	Migraine or tension headaches			
6	Irritable Bowel Syndrome			
7	Multiple Chemical Sensitivities			
8	Neck injury (including whiplash)			
9	Anxiety or panic attacks			
10	Depression			

Reprinted with permission

Our emotions and thoughts have a multiplying effect on our pain. Not only can they worsen our physical experience of the pain, but they also may affect how we respond to the pain and our subsequent suffering. That makes behavioral therapy so important. Behavioral therapy can decrease the negative behavioral and emotional response to the pain and reduce the stimulation of the SS nerves, thus reducing the physical pain as well.

> The therapist can be very important in helping the treatment team to understand the underlying source of the pain and the relative contribution of each type of pain, as many physicians treating pain are unfamiliar with (or completely unaware of) CSP.

When working with individuals with chronic pain, it is important for everyone on the treatment team to understand the underlying source of the pain and the relative contribution of each type of pain. The therapist can be very important in this regard, as many physicians treating pain are unfamiliar with (or completely unaware of) CSP.

OPIOID WITHDRAWAL PAIN

Opioid withdrawal pain is not a chronic pain but may be the leading reason people on long-term opioid medications for the treatment of chronic pain cannot stop their medications. The use of opioids can cause central sensitization and also has many other effects that increase pain on withdrawal of the opioid. For individuals who are addicted to opioids and for those who are on moderate or high doses of opioids for pain, withdrawal usually causes severe pain. Many people with addiction say that the pain from withdrawal is almost unbearable—and many believe that they are going to die. Similarly, attempts at reducing opioid dosage in those who are on long-term opioid medication for the treatment of chronic pain typically result in severe pain. This causes the person to believe that there is no way that they can ever stop taking opioids.

Because of the tolerance that develops to opioids, people may do well when they first start taking them but experience reduced effectiveness after a few months. Tolerance, combined with another phenomenon called **opioid hyperalgesia**, actually makes the pain feel worse until the dosage is increased. People get into a destructive cycle with their doctors, in which they require a higher opioid dosage to get some improvement of pain, but this is followed by worsening pain, requiring ever-increasing dosages. Because withdrawal from opioids makes them feel so much worse, many people try reducing once, feel the pain is too severe, resume opioids, and then never want to stop taking them again.

WHY DO SOME PEOPLE DEVELOP CHRONIC PAIN?

Surprisingly, we don't have a good answer for this question. Obviously, everybody experiences pain in at some point—it is part of the human experience. Why does some acute pain never get better and become chronic? How can we prevent this from happening?

We do know that ongoing pain causes neuroplastic changes to the brain that may lead to the development of central sensitization and chronic pain. Some people may have central sensitization prior to an injury, which may predispose them to a bad outcome.

The severity of an injury does *not* appear to have an effect on the development of chronic pain. Chronic neck pain develops in about one-fourth of those who sustain a whiplash injury in a motor vehicle crash. The severity of the crash or the injury does not make a difference in which people develop chronic pain. However, the person's pre-accident perception of their own health and their coping skills *do* have an impact on the development of chronic pain.

The use of opioids early after trauma may have a calming effect, but their use may also lead to chronic pain. Prescribing opioids early after a workplace back injury doubles the risk of the person developing ongoing pain and disability.

WHAT THERAPISTS NEED TO KNOW

It is important for clinicians to understand their clients' pain and to help them understand their own pain. Knowing *why* they have pain can greatly improve how people with chronic pain live and function. If there is a large component of CSP, the medical provider will not be able to do much to relieve the pain. Shots and surgery will not help, because the pain is originating in areas of the brain that aren't related to physical injury. Similarly, ibuprofen and other anti-inflammatory medications will not help. Opioids may help in the short term but have worse outcomes in the long term. Antidepressants may have some benefit, but behavioral therapy is clearly the treatment of choice.

Key Points to Understanding Pain

- There are **two types of pain**: Acute pain lasts less than 3 months and is normal pain. Chronic pain lasts more than 3 months and is not normal or helpful.

- There are **four mechanisms of pain**: Nociceptive, neuropathic, central sensitization, and opioid withdrawal.

- Almost all acute pain is **nociceptive**. There may also be a CSP component in some people. If CSP is occurring, then the pain is magnified and appears to be out of proportion to the injury.

- Most chronic pain has an element of **CSP**. Pain in conditions such as fibromyalgia, chronic back pain, and chronic daily headaches is almost all CSP.

- **Chronic pain without CSP** is usually mild to moderate and well tolerated. It is also not very common, as most chronic pain has an element of CSP.

Assessing Pain

> *"In boxing, you get hit, it's painful, then you sit on the stool when the adrenaline is gone and you feel that pain. And then you fight the next round."*
>
> —Ben Horowitz

Let's talk about how chronic pain impacts people. It's important to look at both the physical and the psychological cycles of chronic pain.

In the illustration that follows, you can see how both psychological and physical components play a part in how people experience chronic pain. The psychological component of pain is critically important because it leads to both depression and increased pain; it also directly activates the somatosensory nerves when there is a component of central sensitization.

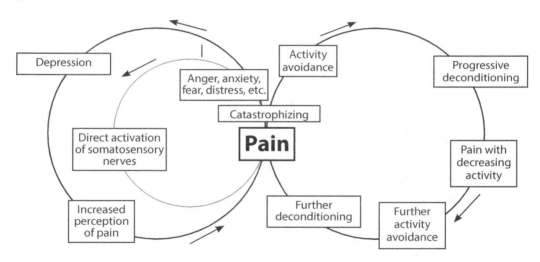

Psychological pain component   **Physical pain component**

Some of the psychological factors involved in chronic pain are anger, anxiety, fear, and distress, which can lead to low mood, depression, and an increased perception of pain. These psychological factors also directly activate the somatosensory nerves causing pain. This cycle can spiral down, compounding both pain and suffering.

Coupled with those psychological features is the physical aspect of the chronic pain cycle. People who have chronic pain commonly experience activity avoidance. This can happen because of anxiety and fear of movement; they're afraid that movement will worsen their pain or that it will cause further damage.

> People with chronic pain often fear movement because they're afraid that it will worsen their pain or that it will cause further damage.

Limited activity leads to physical deconditioning. People become more sedentary, which contributes to loss of strength and muscle mass. They are less likely to exercise regularly or to be as active as they used to be. With deconditioning, people develop balance problems, are more likely to fall, and may be at increased risk of other physical problems like obesity, metabolic syndrome, diabetes, heart disease, and lung disease.

Deconditioning can also have the unintended consequence of increasing pain due to decreased activity. Ironically, this can lead to even more activity avoidance, which only makes the deconditioning worse. It becomes an endless loop.

The cycle of chronic pain ends up feeling like a trap that is nearly impossible to escape. For many people, this leads to hopelessness, pessimism, and despair.

As we consider how chronic pain intrudes on people's lives, we should look at the psychological, behavioral, social, and physical aspects. Let's consider the following example of how chronic pain impacts Maria in all those areas.

Case Example

MARIA – FEARING PAIN

Maria is a 37-year-old mother of three. She comes to you because her doctor suggested it. *"I don't know what good this is going to do. I've seen shrinks before and it never helped. What I really need is a doctor who can finally figure out why I hurt all the time and make it stop,"* she says as she sighs heavily. When asked about what's going on for her, she describes a long pattern of pain:

"I guess it started when I began having my period. I had horrible cramps and could hardly stand the pain. My doctor gave me pain pills, but they eventually stopped working, even though I was taking more and more of them. I started to dread having my period and knew it would be as bad as usual, but sometimes the pain was even worse. I couldn't do anything when the pain was bad, and I stayed home in bed more. I felt like I'd have pain all my life."

She tears up as she continues, *"Nobody has been able to help me, so now I'm thinking this will never get better. I'm getting out less, I'm depressed, I dread my next period, and now my belly hurts all the time, not only during my period."*

PSYCHOLOGICAL ASPECT

When we talk about the psychological component of chronic pain, we are focusing on the thoughts and emotions that people have about their pain. Most people fear pain. This usually develops out of an experience with pain, either acute or chronic. Think about a time that you had acute pain. Maybe you smashed your thumb with a hammer or fell down some steps and sprained your ankle. A natural response would be to have greater fear the next time you use a hammer or go down the stairs where you fell. You are probably going to be more careful and aware of the risk and want to avoid repeating that painful experience.

Along with fearing pain, a lot of people develop anxiety about it. They may start to anticipate it with a dose of apprehension and nervousness. Folks with chronic pain may become keenly aware of signals in their body that may be signs of impending, but not current, pain. That fear can develop into hyperawareness of the *possibility* of the onset of pain, even when it is not happening in the moment. As you may guess, this can become consuming.

One of the essential things to consider when looking at the psychological experience of pain is the negative thought patterns that people develop. These persistent negative thoughts often contribute to the pain experience.

People often develop fear around causing further injury or doing something that increases their level of pain. This may happen when people view pain as proof that they are damaging their bodies rather than seeing pain as a relatively stable problem that could improve. When this fear of harm is greater, people tend to report higher pain intensity.

Pain catastrophizing is a major part of the chronic pain experience. Catastrophizing occurs when people's thoughts jump to the worst possible things that could happen. This type of thinking involves a bigger, more dramatic response than is warranted, and it happens to the majority of people with chronic pain. Let's say that you wake up in the middle of the night in pain...again. Maybe you have another headache. If you have a tendency to catastrophize, you might be alarmed and tell yourself:

> *This keeps happening! This is only going to get worse. I may have to call in sick to work tomorrow. I probably won't be able to go back to sleep, and I'll be exhausted all day tomorrow. Nothing helps these headaches. I don't know why the doctors can't fix this. I've tried everything. I'll never get better. Maybe this is a brain tumor!*

Can you see how catastrophizing can actually make your pain worse (and disrupt your sleep)? Chronic pain can become consuming. It can control people's lives and become a primary focus of attention. It's easy to see how this can happen. Imagine that you have chronic pain in some area of your body, maybe low back pain. After having this pain for a while, you start to pay more attention to your lower back and any signs that the pain is getting worse. You mentally check in on your back several times throughout the day (and night). Is it hurting more? Is there tension in your back? Are you noticing any sharp pains? Cramping? Pain with movement? It can be hard to think of much else when you spend so much time thinking about your back pain. This hypervigilance can make pain worse instead of better.

Sometimes pain becomes so intense that people think they could die from it. People may even think that death could bring release from their pain, but they still feel a fear of dying. Pain itself doesn't kill people; diseases, injuries, and various conditions may cause death, but pain alone doesn't. Helping people remember that can help bring a greater sense of perspective when they are in pain.

Other common psychological components of chronic pain are anxiety and depression. Pain and depression commonly coexist. About two-thirds of people with depression also have chronic pain, and as many as 85% of people with chronic pain have depression. Dealing with the long-term frustration of chronic pain can certainly wear people down and contribute to a sense of despair or defeat. Things may seem hopeless, and people may feel they've tried everything and seen many professionals with no relief from their pain. They may not be sleeping well, they hurt a lot, and they're less active. It can seem like a setup for depressive or anxious symptoms. Remember that hopelessness, anxiety, depression and other mood disorders magnify pain through central sensitization.

> Pain and depression commonly coexist. About two-thirds of people with depression also have chronic pain, and as many as 85% of people with chronic pain have depression.

Sometimes people cope in ways that aren't helpful and actually make pain worse. People may overeat, drink too much, withdraw, get angry, or become less active. There are many coping tactics that end up adding to pain rather than reducing it.

People with chronic pain may develop a "sick role" and see themselves as chronically sick or in pain. Their identity may shift to a situation in which they no longer view themselves as productive or contributing to their families or society at large. This change in self-image can be damaging and often adds to the person's perception of pain.

Another way that psychology impacts the pain experience occurs when people don't have a clearly diagnosed cause for the pain. They'll often seek answers, and when none are given, pain is seen as a mystery, which leads to more distress and greater pain intensity. This can block the effective management of pain.

BEHAVIORAL ASPECT

There are several ways that chronic pain affects people behaviorally. Chronic pain can begin to control people's lives and lead them to withdraw from their normal activities, hobbies, and interests. As was mentioned previously, people who used to be physically active become less so. The discomfort they feel when they are moving around can lead them to move around less. This reduced activity level dramatically

> Chronic pain can begin to control people's lives and lead them to withdraw from their normal activities, hobbies, and interests.

changes their lifestyles. People with chronic pain often find that they are less involved in hobbies and interests than they once were and they often reduce their involvement in pleasurable activities. All of these behavioral changes lead to a lower quality of life.

These very common side effects of chronic pain are areas that behavioral treatment can directly target. This can make a big difference. For example, helping people increase their involvement in pleasant activities is a powerful intervention.

SOCIAL ASPECT

People with chronic pain often report that their social lives have taken a huge hit. Intimate relationships with partners, family members, and friends may become frayed. Struggles in the relationship with a partner may lead to increased pain. Partners may be overly solicitous or helpful, increasing the dependence and helplessness of the person with chronic pain. On the other hand, when a person has chronic pain, their partner may become distant or punishing and grow weary of hearing about the pain concerns. Having a solicitous or punitive partner doesn't do anything to help the person in pain.

Relatives may become frustrated and feel that family dynamics revolve around the person with chronic pain. Family plans may change based on how that person is feeling at the time. Normal family activities may not happen the way that they used to. Relatives may also contribute to the sick role described earlier by protecting their loved one with pain and enabling them to reduce activity instead of increasing it.

> Partners may be overly solicitous or helpful, increasing the dependence and helplessness of the person with chronic pain. On the other hand, when a person has chronic pain, their partner may become distant or punishing and grow weary of hearing about the pain concerns.

Friends may start to pull away from the person with chronic pain. Social activities may be planned only to have the person cancel at the last minute if they are having a bad day. Friends may not know how to respond to the emotional needs of the person with chronic pain and may feel at a loss about how to offer support.

The social impact can damage work relationships as well. Coworkers and supervisors may feel resentful or question how bad the person's pain *really* is. People with chronic pain may need more time off to go to various appointments or may need work accommodations, both of which can lead to stress in workplace relationships.

All of these social changes may lead to further deconditioning, sadness, withdrawal, low mood, worthlessness, and further social isolation.

PHYSICAL ASPECT

As we look at the areas in which people experience pain, we also need to consider the physical realm. Obviously, *pain hurts*. Few of us enjoy pain, look forward to it, or welcome it. Far from it!

Our first instinct is to protect what hurts and rest it. That is an important behavioral response for acute pain, as it may be necessary for the injury to heal. However, chronic pain is different. Resting may be the least helpful thing people can do, although it's often their first instinct. They may develop protective movement patterns that can cause discomfort in the body because posture becomes crooked, they are walking with a limp, or they are not using certain muscles. Guarding, limping, bracing, and not using the painful part of the body contribute to greater pain. Becoming less active and more sedentary can add to the risk of the person developing other conditions, which makes them hurt more and feel greater discomfort.

> People with chronic pain often report that they view their bodies differently. They may feel betrayed by their bodies when they no longer do what they want them to do.

People with chronic pain often report that they view their bodies differently. They may feel betrayed by their bodies when they no longer do what they want them to do. Rather than feeling strong and capable, they may feel weak and vulnerable. Instead of trusting their bodies to work well, they no longer feel that confident optimism. Maybe you've experienced a similar feeling when your car suddenly develops problems and only starts some of the time. You no longer have that blind faith that your car will do what it's always done for you in the past. Imagine feeling that way about your own body.

The following worksheet is designed to help people with chronic pain assess the various ways that pain has affected them. Use this tool to help your clients look at how chronic pain affects them psychologically, behaviorally, socially, and physically.

Assessing Pain's Impact

Please take some time to think about the impact that living with chronic pain has on you. Carefully considering your responses can help you target the areas in which you are most impacted.

Understanding your own experience with pain can guide you as you begin treatment. As you identify the psychological, behavioral, social, and physical consequences of living with chronic pain, you will be able to move forward with a greater sense of direction and purpose.

How does your pain impact you **psychologically** (thoughts and emotions)?

_____

_____

_____

How does your pain affect you **behaviorally**?

_____

_____

_____

How does your pain impact you **socially**?

_____

_____

_____

How does your pain affect you **physically**?

_____

_____

_____

Key Points to Assessing Pain

- **The chronic pain cycle** is a map of both physical and psychological components.

- The **psychological component** leads to depression and increased pain; it also directly activates the somatosensory nerves for people with central sensitization.

- The **physical aspect** of the chronic pain cycle leads to activity avoidance and deconditioning. The unintended consequence of this may be weakness and physical illness.

- People with chronic pain are impacted **behaviorally**. They may be less involved in activities and hobbies and have a poorer quality of life.

- The **social component** of chronic pain contributes to isolation, relationship struggles, and work challenges.

- While the **physical aspect** of pain may be the most obvious, it should be noted that people change their body movements and develop maladaptive physical coping mechanisms.

Trauma and Pain

> *"Pain is real when you get other people to believe it.*
> *If no one believes in it but you, your pain is madness or hysteria."*
> —*Naomi Wolf*

It is well established that the emotional aspect of pain is often more problematic than the physical aspect. Chronic pain includes both physical and emotional components that can't be separated from each other.

The following pie chart provides a visual representation of how much of a role thoughts and emotions play in chronic pain compared with in acute pain. As you can see, thoughts and emotions play a much more significant part in chronic pain. It's imperative that we address these components as key contributors to chronic pain.

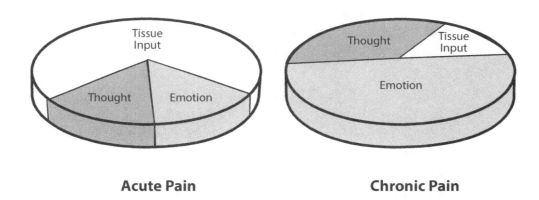

Acute Pain   **Chronic Pain**

Emotional distress leads to worse outcomes following surgery and hospitalizations. People who feel more emotional upset prior to surgery have consistently poorer postsurgical results. They report greater pain intensity, use more opioid pain medication, have significantly more functional impairment, and take longer to recover.

The evidence shows that postoperative pain intensity is worse with pain catastrophizing, rumination about pain, and feelings of helplessness in managing pain. People who magnify pain prior to surgery don't do as well after surgery. Depression before surgery is an additional risk factor for worse outcomes after operations of all types.

OUR THOUGHTS AND EXPECTATIONS AFFECT PAIN

Darnall (2014) reports on a fascinating study done in the United Kingdom by Dr. Irene Tracy and others that shows the powerful impact our expectations about pain have on our experience of it. Study participants had intravenous (IV) catheters inserted in their arms and were placed in a functional magnetic resonance imaging (fMRI) machine. They were given a painful stimulus that they rated an average of 66 out of 100 on a pain scale. Without knowing it, they were given a strong opioid through the IV. Their pain only dropped to a 55.

When the researchers told the participants they would be given a strong opioid through the IV, the pain dropped to an average of 35, even though the medication had actually *never been administered*. It was the *expectation* of pain relief that brought a reduction in pain, not the actual medication. This is the **placebo effect**. A reduction in pain occurs because of an individual's expectation that the treatment will help even when it does not do anything physiological.

> It was the *expectation* of pain relief that brought a reduction in pain, not the actual medication. This is the **placebo effect.**

> The **nocebo effect** happens when pain is increased because of a person's expectations of worse pain.

Next, the study participants were told that the opioid would be stopped (though it wasn't). Their average pain intensity quickly jumped up to a 64—almost the same as their initial pain rating, even though *they were still receiving the IV opioid*. This is called the **nocebo effect**. This happens when pain is increased because of a person's expectations of worse pain.

What does this tell us? It's our *expectation* of pain that causes misery, not the physical sensations of pain. Our brains cause pain more than our bodies do.

Another study (Benedetti et al., 2002) reported similar findings. Participants were set up with IV lines in their arms while they experienced pain. Pain was reduced when morphine was administered through the IV from outside the room, but pain decreased more dramatically when a staff member came into the room and administered it in full view of the study participants. When a saline placebo was put in the IV from outside the room, it had no effect on pain but when given in front of the participant, a reduction in pain was reported.

Another study (Levine & Gordon, 1984) looked at dental patients who had a molar removed. They were each given a placebo saline injection with the suggestion that it was a potent painkiller. This "fake" shot was as effective in relieving their pain as 6 to 8 mg of morphine.

One more example of the power of our expectations has to do with the cold pressor test. The cold pressor test involves a person placing a hand into an ice water bath and indicating when they first feel pain; participants are instructed not to remove their hand from the ice water until the pain is unbearable. **Pain threshold** is the point at which sensation becomes pain, and **pain tolerance** is the total length of time the hand stays in the icy bath minus the threshold time.

A few unexpected findings are worth noting. People on opioids actually have *lower* pain tolerance during the cold pressor test due to opioid hyperalgesia. The other curious result is that if people simply handle a bottle of ibuprofen between two cold pressor tests, their pain tolerance is increased in the second test. They didn't *take* any ibuprofen; they merely handled the bottle. Finally, pain tolerance decreases when people believe they will have to keep their hand in the icy bath for a long period of time. Pain tolerance increases when they believe the discomfort will be short-lived.

Goldstein and colleagues (2016) published a study that demonstrated the pain-reducing properties of empathetic touch for women in labor. They found that when the woman's partner touched her with empathy, her pain was dramatically reduced. Interestingly, this finding was noticed only if the partner felt empathy toward the laboring partner *during the time the touching took place.* There was no pain reduction when a partner touched without feeling empathy. The findings were not the same when an empathetic stranger touched the laboring woman. The touch of a stranger, even one with empathy, did not produce the same pain reduction. The greater the empathy felt by the touching partner, the greater the pain relief. This offers striking evidence of pain reduction related to receiving emotionally empathetic partner touch.

These results offer further evidence of the power of the mind in the pain experience. We're so used to expecting pain pills to be helpful that pain is actually reduced just by the expectation—even in the absence of actual pain medication. As these studies show, there are numerous ways in which our thoughts and feelings impact our experience of pain.

EMOTIONS THAT INCREASE PAIN

There are several factors that increase the amount of pain and suffering that people with chronic pain endure. Most of these factors are emotional and not determined by actual damage to tissue. They augment and magnify pain through central sensitization.

People often feel **anger** about the amount of pain they have and length of time they've had it. They may be angry at themselves, their doctors, or their families. Anger can extend toward the "system" for not being helpful enough or toward God or another higher power when they feel that life is unfair and they are not getting adequate relief.

> People with chronic pain become keenly aware of their bodies and the discomfort that they feel. They can develop an apprehensive awareness of bodily cues and may be on the lookout for any indicators that pain is building.

Pain is a stress reaction and arouses **fear** for most people with frequent pain. The fear may be related to never getting relief from the pain and not being able to return to prior functioning and wellness. The fear of a future filled with pain can be overwhelming. Constantly looking for a solution and finding none feeds fear.

Chronic pain often leads to **anxiety**. People become keenly aware of their bodies and the discomfort that they feel. They can develop an apprehensive awareness of bodily cues and may be on the lookout for any indicators that pain is building.

Depression is often coupled with chronic pain, adding to the ongoing emotional (and physical) upset that people experience. With a low mood comes decreased motivation and less energy to tackle what must be done to rise above constant pain. Depression impacts pain, and pain impacts depression.

The more impacted people are by the emotional aspect of pain, the greater their suffering. We often see that their thoughts are becoming more problematic. With increased suffering comes stronger aversive thoughts and **pessimism**. This negative mindset contributes to the agitation that people feel as they lose a sense of control over their situation and feel ineffective in managing their pain. Pain becomes a consuming experience—one that people may try with all their might to get rid of with no success. The wish for relief becomes so compelling that it's all they can think of. Ironically, this fervent hope does little to move people from pain to progress. This seems like evidence of failure, which builds frustration and self-punitive thoughts.

Another problematic thought pattern, and one that leads to changes in behavior, is **learned helplessness.** In studies with rats, we see that when they cause pain to themselves by pressing a bar, they eventually stop pressing the bar. However, when rats have pain that they can't control, they act anxious, stressed, and hypervigilant. The rats in that state don't do as well with problems like getting through a maze. They may also withdraw and lose their appetite.

Similarly, people with chronic pain may give up and stop trying to find solutions when they feel they have little control—they don't believe they have the power to stop their pain. This learned helplessness becomes a self-defeating pattern. This is similar to the previously mentioned sick role, in which people with chronic pain adopt a passive and dependent approach to their condition rather than advocating for themselves in a proactive way.

As we consider the emotions that can increase pain let's take a look at James. As you work with people who have chronic pain you may find that they share many similar emotions with James.

Case Example

James – The Impact of Pain

James comes into your office limping with a grimace on his face. He immediately gets down to business, saying:

"I'm just so tired of this. I hurt all the time. I injured my back at work two years ago, and I haven't been the same since. I'm mad at my boss for not believing me and not taking any responsibility for what happened to me. I haven't been able to get disability, which is ridiculous. I feel like the system is out to screw with me."

As he takes a breath, he carefully shifts his position in the chair, saying, *"I'm scared about my finances and not being able to pay my bills. I'm worried about losing my house. This just gets me so down that I don't know how I'm going to go on. It seems like there's nothing I can do and nobody who can help me."*

As suffering increases, you observe more maladaptive postures, nonrestorative breathing patterns, grimacing, wincing, bracing, propping, and other protective movements. All of these behavioral responses actually worsen pain, as they disrupt healthy movement, breathing, and posture.

THE TRAUMA LINK

It's worth noting that childhood trauma contributes to chronic pain in late adolescence and into adulthood. This is demonstrated by the Adverse Childhood Experiences (ACE) Study. A collaboration between the Centers for Disease Control and Kaiser Healthcare, this landmark study was published in 1998. The goal was to look at the lifelong impact of childhood trauma on adult health and well-being. Participants were 17,000 health maintenance organization (HMO) members in Southern California. The questionnaire included 10 questions on childhood trauma, with each positive response being worth one point.

The results are shocking: Participants had scores indicating adverse effects in several areas: physical, behavioral, emotional, social, developmental, financial, and criminal. Even *one* point on the questionnaire raises the risk of chronic pain in adulthood. With a score of four or more, the risk of suicide is 12 times greater. The risk of addiction goes up relative to the number of points a person scores.

The ACE Study provides the clearest evidence yet of the horrific lifelong impact of childhood trauma on chronic pain, addiction, and suicide. A large study by the Centers for Disease Control and Prevention (CDC; Olivieri, 2012) illustrates this in a dramatic way, demonstrating the impact of ACEs in people with fibromyalgia compared with people without it. People with fibromyalgia were shown to have a much greater likelihood of having experienced certain types of trauma in childhood. For example, they were much more likely to have grown up with a depressed person (47%, compared with 15% of healthy control group) and to have experienced physical and verbal abuse by parents (42%, compared with 10% of healthy controls for physical abuse and 53%, compared with 23% for verbal abuse).

When we look at the link between fibromyalgia and sexual trauma the results are also stunning: People who experienced attempted sexual touch by an adult, sexual touch by an adult, or forced sex with an adult represented 21% to 34% of people with fibromyalgia but only 4% to 9% of the healthy sample. Another finding from the CDC study is that ACEs that are specifically targeted against the child (such as abuse) have a greater negative effect than negative events to which the child is exposed but aren't directed toward the child (e.g., parents abusing each other but not the child).

> The ACE Study provides the clearest evidence yet of the horrific lifelong impact of childhood trauma in chronic pain, addiction, and suicide.

The ACE questions are listed in the worksheet that follows. This can be given to clients to complete to help you understand their trauma history. Even a score of one is worth talking about with your clients. You may choose to provide some education to help people understand their scores and the impact of the trauma suffered in childhood.

Adverse Childhood Experiences

During your first 18 years of life . . .

1. Did a parent or other adult in the household often or very often swear at you, insult you, put you down, or humiliate you? Or act in a way that made you afraid that you might be physically hurt?

    Yes   No   (If yes, enter 1 _____)

2. Did a parent or other adult in the household often or very often push, grab, slap, or throw something at you? Or ever hit you so hard that you had marks or were injured?

    Yes   No   (If yes, enter 1 _____)

3. Did an adult or person at least five years older than you ever touch or fondle you or have you touch their body in a sexual way? Or attempt to or actually have oral, anal, or vaginal intercourse with you?

    Yes   No   (If yes, enter 1 _____)

4. Did you often or very often feel that no one in your family loved you or thought you were important or special? Or your family didn't look out for each other, feel close to each other, or support each other?

    Yes   No   (If yes, enter 1 _____)

5. Did you often or very often feel that you didn't have enough to eat, had to wear dirty clothes, or had no one to protect you? Or your parents were too drunk or high to take care of you or take you to the doctor if needed?

    Yes   No   (If yes, enter 1 _____)

6. Were your parents ever separated or divorced?

    Yes   No   (If yes, enter 1 _____)

7. Was your mother or step-mother often or very often pushed, grabbed, slapped, or had something thrown at her? Or sometimes, often, or very often kicked, bitten, hit with a fist, or hit with something hard? Or ever repeatedly hit for at least a few minutes or threatened with a gun or knife?

Yes   No   (If yes, enter 1 _____)

8. Did you live with anyone who was a problem drinker or alcoholic or who used street drugs?

Yes   No   (If yes, enter 1 _____)

9. Was a household member depressed or mentally ill, or did a household member attempt suicide?

Yes   No   (If yes, enter 1 _____)

10. Did a household member go to prison?

Yes   No   (If yes, enter 1 _____)

Now add up your "Yes" answers: _____. This is your ACE Score.

SUICIDE

The risk of suicide in people with chronic pain is real and must be addressed. The statistics on the prevalence of suicide in this population are staggering. Cheatle (2011) studied suicide in people with chronic pain: In this study, up to half of the participants had suicidal ideation. Passive ideation was evident in 19% to 24%, while about 13% had active ideation. About one in 20 had a suicide plan, and 5% had made a previous suicide attempt.

The risk of suicide is clearly higher for people who are pain catastrophizers. Sleep problems, which are common with pain, also raise the risk of suicide. Helplessness and hopelessness contribute as well. The more fervently someone hopes to escape from pain, the greater the risk. People who are avoidant in addressing their pain are also in a high-risk group.

Opioids are particularly problematic when considering the risk of depression and suicide. About 20% of *all* people who die by suicide test positive for opioids. Nearly 75% of people with chronic pain who die by suicide do it by overdosing on opioids. This points to the fact that many people suffering with the misery and despair of chronic pain feel that it is too much to live with, leading to suicidal ideation, attempts, and completion. Science has clearly shown that opioid use only worsens depression and suicidal behavior. Despite these findings, drug manufacturers and their physician spokespeople typically say that the risk of depression and suicide in those with chronic pain is precisely why we should be prescribing more opioids instead of limiting them. These issues make it imperative that behavioral health providers do a thorough suicide risk assessment and regularly assess for suicidal ideation. Working with people to reduce not only their pain but also their suicidal thinking is one of the most important ways we can intervene.

Key Points of Trauma and Pain

- The **emotional aspect** of pain is usually more problematic than the physical aspect. This is more of a factor with chronic pain than with acute pain. These emotions include:

  - Anger
  - Fear
  - Anxiety
  - Depression
  - Pessimism
  - Learned helplessness

- There is often a clear **trauma** link in many people with chronic pain. People with ACE (Adverse Childhood Experience) points are at greater risk of developing chronic pain.
- The risk of **suicide** is much higher in people with chronic pain. Opioid use increases this risk.

Chapter 4

The Illusion of Opioids

> *"And now, my beauties, something with poison in it, I think.*
> *With poison in it, but attractive to the eye and to the smell.*
> *Poppies ... poppies ... poppies will put them to sleep.*
> *Sleeeeep. Now they'll sleeeeep!"*
>
> —*Wicked Witch of the West, The Wizard of Oz*

In the first three chapters, we discussed the physical and emotional aspects of pain. By now, you understand pain better than the great majority of physicians who are treating it. You may also realize that it is a mistake to separate the physical and emotional aspects of pain, because they are so closely integrated. It is also seemingly impossible to separate pain from the impact of opioid use when looking at our societal problem with pain. It is generally considered (though unproven) that opioids are the most effective medications for pain. People expect opioids for pain, and doctors

> The United States is only 4.6% of the world's population, yet we consume 80% of the world's opioids. Why is it that the United States has such a love affair with opioids? To answer that question, it is important to understand the opioid receptor.

prescribe them freely. The United States contains only 4.6% of the world's population, yet we consume 80% of the world's opioids. Why is it that the United States has such a love affair with opioids? To answer that question, it is important to understand the opioid receptor.

THE OPIOID RECEPTOR

Opioid receptors are molecules, or receptor sites, in the body that capture the opioid molecule and begin a cascade of events that result in the physical and psychological processes that help reduce pain. Beyond reducing pain, opioids have many other effects. Knowing these effects helps us understand why opioids have been the most destructive medicines in the history of humankind.

We have billions of opioid receptors throughout our brain and spinal cord. Although the opioid receptor is the reason opioids have any effect at all, most physicians don't know their purpose. That is surprising, given that doctors are prescribing numerous medications that flood this special molecule. The purpose of the opioid receptor is not to relieve pain; it is to help us achieve a goal.

Our opioid receptors are meant to be activated by our own endogenous opioid neuropeptides—**endorphins**. As we consider how this system affects us, think about the "runner's high" that long-distance runners often describe feeling near the end of a race as their own endorphins are released to help them achieve their goal of finishing. This feeling gives runners renewed energy and confidence that they can complete the race.

Activation of our opioid receptors results in:

- Increased motivation
- Heightened confidence
- Renewed energy
- Reduction of any physical pain
- Decreased anxiety and/or depression
- Increased desire for social bonding with others
- Stimulation of dopamine release that results in a pleasurable feeling

You can see that the activation of our opioid receptors results in the factors that we need to be successful. We can look at this as our "success system."

Opioids only lead to a minimal reduction in pain. The other effects they produce are more significant and are often what cause people to become addicted. To better understand our response to the activation of the opioid receptor, let's reflect on a familiar story.

The Wizard of Oz

In the film *The Wizard of Oz,* Dorothy and her friends (the Cowardly Lion, the Tin Man, the Scarecrow) and her dog, Toto, had spent considerable time in the woods on the way to Oz. It was a very dark and scary place for them. They had dealt with apple-throwing trees, the Wicked Witch of the West throwing fire, and wild animals. Worst of all, they never knew what was around the next corner, causing them almost constant fear and anxiety.

There was also an element of sadness and depression for Dorothy, who was missing her family and wanting to get home. The Wicked Witch was trying to stop their progress and get the ruby slippers from Dorothy. As you recall, she did this by placing a field of poppies in front of them as Dorothy and her friends exited the woods.

As they saw the poppies, they had an immediate change of mood and behavior. Instantly, they had increased energy, confidence, and motivation. Oz, the goal, seemed to be just in front of them. They linked arms and began skipping and dancing down the yellow brick road. These behaviors were due to the opium in the poppies flooding their opioid receptors. Massive activation of our "success system" results in a wonderful world where we function at our best.

However, soon Dorothy, Toto, and the Cowardly Lion began to slow down and fall asleep. The Tin Man and the Scarecrow were unaffected, since, as non-mammals, they didn't have opioid receptors. In fact, the Scarecrow didn't even have a brain! You will also remember that the antidote for this drug-induced sleep was snow, sent by Glenda, the Good Witch of the East. When the book on which the film was based was published in 1900,

> *The Wizard of Oz* gives us a peek into the opioid epidemic of the late 1800s and early 1900s.

snow was a nickname for cocaine, just as it is today. Back then, opium was legal and was commonly used in opium dens. When people would consume too much opium and overdose, it would be reversed with cocaine. So, *The Wizard of Oz* gives us a peek into the opioid epidemic of the late 1800s and early 1900s.

Our patients who are seeking treatment for an opioid use disorder may tell us similar stories. They talk about how they had been in very difficult circumstances. Perhaps there was abuse at home. Maybe there was a difficult situation at work or with their relationships. Many people have lived in stressful situations most of their lives.

Their doctors may give them a prescription of Percocet (oxycodone and acetaminophen) for an injury such as an ankle sprain. Suddenly, they feel confident about life. They feel motivated to be good parents, partners, or employees. They have energy. They have almost instant relief of any anxiety or depression that they had suffered. These are powerful and motivating feelings for continued use of opioids even after the physical pain gets better. Most patients will tell us that they did not feel "high." They simply felt like they were better people, so they continued to take the pills.

Unfortunately, these effects don't last long, and individuals need to take more and more to achieve the same feeling. Stopping the medication leads to a rebound that causes them to feel even worse than they did before they started taking it. Just as in *The Wizard of Oz*, the wonderful effect of the opioids does not last; ultimately, continued use of opioids results in a downward spiral of increased emotional and physical pain, and ultimately, addiction.

WHY WE HAVE AN OPIOID PROBLEM

Understanding the opioid receptor helps us to understand why opioids have become such a difficult problem in our society. They do so much more than reduce pain. For many people, opioids give them the energy, hope, and confidence that they have not had for a long time (if ever). Many who have been suffering from chronic pain for an extended time have chronic feelings of despair and depression. For them, the risks involved with starting an opioid are even greater than for others. Their despair immediately turns to happiness and joy because of the emotional effects of the opioids. Unfortunately, as with Dorothy, those effects won't last. The initial joy that individuals with chronic pain experience with opioid use is replaced by renewed despair that can only be overcome by increasing the dosage of the opioid.

In the 1990s, Purdue Pharmaceuticals produced a DVD that was given to medical professionals regarding their premier product, OxyContin (oxycodone). The video showed seven individuals who had been suffering from chronic pain. They talked at length about how the pain was destroying their lives. However, they claimed, once they started on OxyContin, their lives were transformed. The DVD showed these patients walking, dancing, laughing, and living life to its fullest. They were all experiencing their own "Dorothy reactions." An investigative report 15 years later found that three of the seven individuals had either died from overdose or were actively addicted to opioids.

The "Dorothy reaction" may not be problematic only in those with chronic pain. Opioids may cause this reaction in people with the following conditions, for which opioid therapy should rarely, if ever, be used:

- Depression
- Anxiety
- Bipolar disorder
- Other mental illnesses
- A history of ACEs
- Recent or past emotional trauma
- Family history of addiction
- Personal history of addiction (including tobacco use)

Case Example

Stephen: A Typical Story

Stephen comes to you as a new client with depression and chronic back pain. Nothing in life seems fun anymore. Six months ago, the doctor gave him a prescription for an opioid pain medication. Immediately he felt much better with an elevation in mood as well as a slight reduction in pain. Because of this elevated mood and "Dorothy reaction," life seemed dramatically better. Four weeks later, he returned to his doctor and told her that she is the best medical provider he's ever seen. The medication was continued.

After three to four months, the mood-elevating effects wore off, and tolerance to the pain-relieving properties developed. Stephen went back to the doctor. He told the doctor that the medication worked great for several months, but now his pain is getting worse. His doctor increased the dosage. Once again, he had dramatic improvement in both mood and physical function. This time, the improvement only lasted one or two months, so again, he returned to his physician. By this time, significant physical tolerance had developed. His brain had also developed permanent changes that caused him to experience increased anxiety, depression, and pain.

An attempt to stop the medication after being on it for three months resulted in dramatic worsening of his physical and emotional condition. This made discontinuation of the medication almost impossible. Stephen now sincerely believes that the medication is absolutely necessary for him to function and live. At this point, weaning off the medication will be difficult. People on long-term opioids have greater incidence of depression and anxiety. They also have a worse quality of life. Studies have shown that although weaning off opioids at this point is extremely difficult, those who successfully do it experience approximately a 20% decrease in pain.

Because of the way opioids work on the brain, people with a significant amount of CSP are likely to have increased activation of the brain's somatosensory nerves. When you combine this effect with the hyperalgesia caused by opioids and the pain that occurs on opioid withdrawal, these drugs become very risky for anyone with CSP as a primary component of their chronic pain syndrome. That is why the American Academy of Neurology has said that the risk from opioids is almost always greater than any benefit for those with chronic back pain, fibromyalgia, or chronic headaches (Franklin, 2014).

OPIOIDS FOR ACUTE PAIN ARE ALSO PROBLEMATIC

Chronic pain is not the only situation where the mood-elevating effects of the opioids are problematic. Even when used for acute pain, they can be dangerous in those with risk factors. A common scenario we see is when opioids have been prescribed by an obstetrician to a woman after childbirth. Coming home with a new baby is always a stressful time, and hormonal changes make women more susceptible to feelings of depression. Sometimes the stress of taking care of the new baby can be almost overwhelming to a young woman.

When new mothers take opioid pain medication, they suddenly have a surge of confidence, energy, and mood that is very powerful. They find they can get more accomplished as they care for their baby. Studies have shown that because of these properties of opioids, use to treat acute pain even for just seven days can delay recovery, increase medical costs, and double the risk of future disability. Considering these problems, opioids should only be used for very short periods of time and only when necessary.

> Studies have shown that because of the powerful properties of opioids, use to treat acute pain even for just seven days can delay recovery, increase medical costs, and double the risk of future disability.

The CDC has shown that even a one-day prescription for an opioid for acute pain results in a 6% chance that the individual will still be on it a year later. If that prescription is for eight days, then the chance of long-term opioid use goes up to 13.5%. The longer someone is on opioids for acute pain, the worse the prognosis becomes. People on opioids for one year are unlikely to ever get off of them.

CURRENT OPIOID PRESCRIBING PATTERNS

Because of the powerful properties of opioids and aggressive marketing by the pharmaceutical industry, we began to see a tremendous increase in the use of these medications beginning in the mid-1990s. In 1997, we were prescribing enough opioids to provide every man, woman, and child with the equivalent of 96 mg of morphine per year. By 2007, our prescribing had increased to where we could provide the equivalent of more than 700 mg of morphine to every person in the United States. This is equal to 140 Vicodin tablets per person per year.

Primary care doctors and pain specialists commonly prescribe opioids for chronic pain despite the fact that there is *no evidence* that supports their use for this purpose. The belief that opioids work for chronic pain comes from their calming effect, not their pain-relieving properties. Studies have shown that physicians tend to prescribe opioids based on the emotional distress of their patient more than on the numerical pain score.

EFFECTIVENESS

There are few scientific studies that compare the use of oral opioids to oral nonopioid pain medications. For new opioids to be approved by the Food and Drug Administration (FDA), they simply must be shown to be better than placebo. In one recent study investigating the effectiveness of tapentadol (a newer opioid medication), scientists compared all doses of the drug to morphine (60 mg by mouth) and ibuprofen 400 mg. This study found that the most effective medication was ibuprofen. The equivalent of two over-the-counter ibuprofen pills relieved acute pain better than 60 mg of morphine or any dose of tapentadol. Other recent studies have shown that ibuprofen is equal to or better at relieving acute pain than morphine for children recovering from tonsillectomy or fracture (Poonai et al., 2014). There are other studies with similar results—oral opioids are less effective than ibuprofen and similar drugs for relieving pain—and opioids are much more dangerous.

The Cochrane organization evaluation for effectiveness of pain relief looks at how often a medication reduces pain by 50% (e.g., reducing pain from an eight to a four or better on a pain scale). Cochrane studies have examined the treatment of acute pain immediately following surgery.

As you can see in the following graph, one over-the-counter 200mg ibuprofen pill is as effective at relieving pain as two Percocet tablets. Acetaminophen (Tylenol) by itself is better than oxycodone. The combination of one ibuprofen (200mg) and one acetaminophen (500 mg) is better (by far) than all the other options listed.

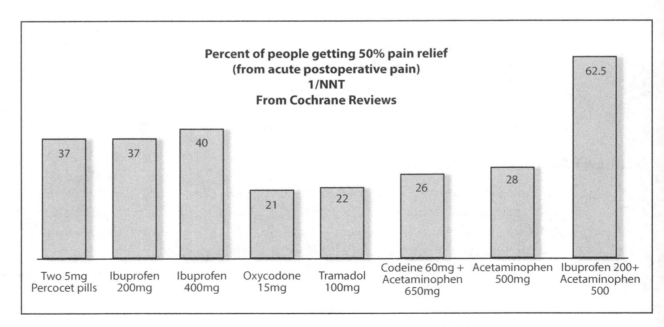

(Christopher Derry et al., 2009; CJ Derry et al., 2013; Gaskell, Derry, Moore, & McQuay, 2009; Moore et al., 2011; Laurence Toms et al., 2008) Reprinted with permission.

The combination of one ibuprofen (200 mg) and one acetaminophen (500 mg) is better (by far) than other medications studied.

For chronic pain, the evidence for opioids is no better. There are no studies that show the effectiveness of opioids beyond 16 weeks of therapy. The short-term studies that have been done show limited effectiveness—usually *less than one point* on a pain scale of 0 to 10. After 16 weeks, patients develop tolerance to the medications, which makes them even less effective. The following graph from a pharmaceutical industry–sponsored study showed that tapentadol reduced chronic pain less than one point compared with placebo and that controlled-release oxycodone (OxyContin) was even less effective.

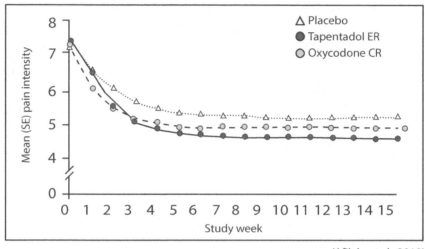

(Afilalo et al., 2010)

Several studies have looked at very large populations of people with chronic pain and have shown that those treated with opioids have a worse quality of life than those with chronic pain who are not on opioids. How can this be? This happens because, as previously noted, opioids cause changes in the brain that lead to *increased* pain, depression, anxiety, and addiction. One key change is in our own opioid system. With ongoing use of opioids, our body reacts by decreasing our opioid receptors and endorphins. With the loss or dysfunction of

Opioids cause changes in the brain that lead to *increased* pain, depression, anxiety, and addiction.

this system, we are no longer motivated to be successful. Excitement and motivation are now replaced by fear and trepidation. We no longer want to do anything. Our pain and our pain pills consume us.

So, what works for chronic pain? As mentioned previously, behavioral therapy is likely the best treatment option to reduce the emotional and physical aspects of pain. Exercise, physical therapy, yoga, and other modalities can help as well. Nonopioid medications have some role, but that role is minor and those medications should be used only after individuals are engaged in behavioral and physical therapy. It is important for clients to understand that medications are not the answer to chronic pain and that the true answer lies within themselves.

SIDE EFFECTS

Opioid pain medications not only are the least effective oral pain medication but also cause the most side effects. Ironically, prescribers often use opioids because they are concerned about the side effects of nonsteroidal anti-inflammatory drugs (NSAIDs) and acetaminophen. It is well known that NSAIDs can cause stomach ulcers and kidney damage when used for prolonged periods. Acetaminophen can cause liver damage when used at higher doses. These problems can be life-threatening when severe, and physicians have seen many patients with these adverse effects. Fortunately, these adverse effects can be easily diagnosed with an examination and simple blood work.

Opioid side effects are different. They are more subtle and often not noticed by physicians. They are also deadlier. More than 30,000 people die each year from the side effects of opioids. This compares with about 3,200 deaths per year from NSAIDs (Tarone, Blot, & McLaughlin, 2004) and about 200 from acetaminophen (Centers for Disease Control and Prevention, National Center for Health Statistics, 2016).

> More than 30,000 people die each year from the side effects of opioids. This compares with about 3,200 deaths per year from NSAIDs and about 200 from acetaminophen.

Hyperalgesia

It is important for us to feel pain. Pain is a defense mechanism that helps us survive. Our brains are incredibly complex organs that change when exposed to opioids. With the first dose of an opioid, our brains immediately begin to compensate to help us feel pain more intensely to overcome the drug's numbing effect. With the initiation of opioid treatment, the brain reduces the availability of the opioid receptor. With ongoing opioid use, our bodies reduce the number of opioid receptors and change the connections of the brain's nerve cells to help us feel pain more intensely. With less availability of the opioid receptor, any opioids taken have a weaker effect, as do our endorphins, resulting in an increased pain sensation. This phenomenon, mentioned previously, is called **opioid hyperalgesia**. It likely occurs in everyone who takes opioids. The result is increased pain as people try to come off opioids. It may be the major reason people with chronic pain have a very hard time stopping opioids after starting on them.

Because of opioid hyperalgesia and withdrawal effects when stopping chronic opioid therapy, the pain *always* gets worse. It may get a lot worse. Because of this, most people feel that they must remain on their opioids. The pills "must be helping" if the pain gets worse when they try to reduce their dose. However, the increase in pain is only temporary (although it may last a few months). Studies show that when people on chronic opioids for chronic pain stop them, there will be an initial period of worsening, and then their pain will improve by an average of 20%.

Brain Effects

To understand other effects that opioids have on the brain, it is important to understand two critical brain processes; the release of dopamine and the activation of the opioid receptor. Both of these processes are critical to our survival.

Dopamine is the "feel-good" chemical of the brain. It is what we live for. Dopamine release is what causes us to feel good when we eat a delicious meal, have sex, or achieve something significant. It is the primary reward chemical that motivates us to survive. Dopamine release is also the ultimate action of all addicting drugs and activities. It's what makes them addicting.

As described earlier, our own opioid system (endorphins and opioid receptors) is our "success system," and activation of the opioid receptor results in several processes that help us achieve a goal. With activation, we feel confidence, energy, hope, a reduced feeling of anxiety and depression, and a feeling of camaraderie with others. We also feel pleasure because dopamine has been released.

Activation of the opioid receptor and stimulation of dopamine are important processes in our bodies that help us survive and be productive. Unfortunately, these systems were designed to work with endogenous opioids (endorphins), not opioid drugs. When we flood our bodies with high levels of unnatural opioids, we initially feel much better, with less pain and more hope, motivation, and happiness. However, as noted, our bodies quickly respond by decreasing opioid receptors; dopamine release also decreases. Over time, people taking opioids daily find themselves feeling the opposite of how they did when they started on the opioids. They have less energy, motivation, confidence, joy, and pleasure.

Our brains adapt in other ways as well. Our brain cells actually change their connections and reroute signals to reinforce the rewards from opioids and decrease connections to the front part of our brain, which is responsible for rational thought. This occurs in all addictions and explains why those with this disease often make decisions in an effort to obtain the substance to which they are addicted that do not seem rational.

Younger and colleagues (2011) studied people with chronic back pain. The researchers treated half of them with ibuprofen and half with morphine. They did an MRI on each patient at the start of treatment and repeated

> Opioids cause brain changes that are likely permanent after just one month of treatment.

it one month later. The researchers could measure changes in different parts of the brains of those taking morphine. Realizing that the opioids were causing brain changes, the researchers immediately stopped the morphine and put all of the patients on ibuprofen. They repeated the MRIs six months later and discovered that the changes were still there. Their conclusion was that opioids cause brain changes that are likely permanent after just one month of treatment.

Impairment

Opioids cause impairments to functioning. This is problematic on our roads and in the workplace. In a review of all studies that had looked at driving impairment and drugs, it was found that the use of opioids by a driver doubles the risk of an accident that results in injury or death (Elvik, 2013).

Impairment is also problematic at work. Most drug-free workplace policies include drug testing designed to identify illicit drug use. If an employee has a positive drug test for opioids but has a prescription from a physician, the test is considered negative. However, the use of opioids is not appropriate for those working in safety-sensitive positions. It also may not be appropriate for those driving to and from work.

Depression

Opioids have a very interesting effect on our mood. The initial doses act as potent antidepressants. In fact, opioids are probably the most effective antidepressant available, successfully treating even those for whom all other treatments for depression have failed. The "Dorothy reaction" is great for those with depression. Unfortunately, that effect does not last. The mood-elevating effects become less and less with each dose, and when the opioid wears off, the person's mood is even *worse* than it was before the opioid was initially taken. For many people on chronic opioid therapy, the best they feel (right after taking their opioid dose) is worse than how they felt before starting on opioids. That is the primary reason that people with chronic pain who are on opioids have twice the rate of depression as those with chronic pain who are not on opioids.

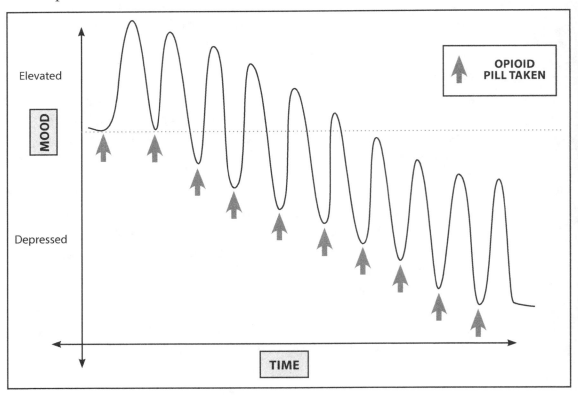

Loss of Pleasure

Even if people taking opioids don't develop depression, they often experience anhedonia, the loss of pleasure in things they used to enjoy. This emotional numbing occurs because of the decreased number of opioid receptors and dysfunction of the opioid system. While this is certainly problematic for the individual taking opioids, it can also be difficult for family and friends. The person can't share in the joy and excitement of family events or vacations. They just don't seem to care.

Drug Interactions

In people taking opioids, drug interactions are a leading cause of unintentional death. Benzodiazepines are particularly deadly when taken with opioids. Many people on opioids have anxiety disorders and are also long-term benzodiazepine users. The CDC guidelines for the use of opioids in chronic pain recommend against using these two medications together. Alcohol and all other sedating drugs also increase the risk of death when taken with opioids and should be avoided.

Death

Taking opioids increases the risk of death by 50% during active use. Unintended overdose is the most obvious cause of death, but death can also occur due to falls and fractures, motor vehicle or

> Taking opioids increases the risk of death by 50% during active use.

work accidents, heart arrhythmias, drug interactions, sleep apnea, immune system suppression, and other problems.

Sleep Problems

Opioids often contribute to sleep problems. They disrupt sleep architecture, making sleep less restorative. When taking opioids, it takes longer to fall asleep, it is harder to stay asleep, and sleep quality is worse. When we sleep, our breathing is regulated by the amount of carbon dioxide (CO_2) in our blood. If we breathe too slowly, the CO_2 builds up, and the brain senses this, making us breathe faster to get rid of the CO_2. Opioids reduce the function of this respiratory control. That is very dangerous in someone with sleep apnea, which causes people to stop breathing until their elevated CO_2 suddenly stimulates their breathing again. Alterations to this regulatory system by the taking of opioids can result in life-threatening complications.

Worse Medical Care

A 2015 study by Gautam and coworkers showed that people on chronic opioid therapy receive worse general care for other medical problems; it also showed that their medical care gets even worse with higher doses of opioids (Gautam, Franzini, Mikhail, Chan, & Turner, 2015). A primary reason for this is that doctors don't feel comfortable treating chronic pain with opioids; therefore, such treatment consumes a lot of the physician's emotional and intellectual energy, leaving less energy for the rest of the patient's medical needs (Jamison et al., 2015).

Constipation

Constipation is experienced to some degree by most people on opioids. While this is not usually life threatening, constipation can reduce quality of life. There are now prescription medications specially designed to treat constipation caused by opioids. This is one of the only areas in medicine where we have a prescription medication solely to treat the side effects of another prescription medication.

Diversion

Unfortunately, no matter how careful we are, many opioids ultimately end up being taken for "nonmedical" reasons. Any use of a medication for which it was not originally intended is considered nonmedical. Nonmedical use is very common. Most people who receive an opioid prescription do not take all of them; about 60% of these patients save some of the pills in their medicine cabinet for later (nonmedical) use. Up to 23% of all opioids prescribed are diverted for nonmedical use.

> Up to one-third of people who take opioids daily for chronic pain will become addicted.

Addiction

Addiction is a destructive brain disease that affects millions of people. Two million people are addicted to opioids in the United States, and more are becoming addicted every day. Addiction is the result of brain changes that occur from taking opioids. It doesn't matter if you are taking them as prescribed or not; up to one-third of people who take opioids daily for chronic pain will become addicted. Addiction to opioids is now called Opioid Use Disorder (OUD). OUD is a fatal disease unless treated.

> Opioids are probably the least effective treatment for acute or chronic pain and have the most side effects of all treatments.

Some people with OUD are successfully treated with counseling and group support (e.g., Narcotics Anonymous). However, about 90% with OUD have permanent brain changes that result in the depression, anxiety, craving, and other symptoms described previously. These people will ultimately relapse unless given medication to help treat this disease. Methadone and Suboxone (buprenorphine with naloxone) are two medications that treat OUD. These medications are not "substituting one addiction for another," as many people say. They work effectively in the brain to control the disease. In fact, when used appropriately, these medications are so successful that individuals taking them will meet NONE of the 11 criteria for OUD.

Hormonal Dysfunction

Opioids have adverse effects on our hormonal systems. Testosterone levels have been shown to decrease four hours after an opioid dose. Ongoing use leads to a chronic decrease in testosterone levels in men and estrogen in women. This results in decreased libido, fatigue, and erectile dysfunction in men. Women experience decreased libido and menstrual irregularities and are at higher risk for osteoporosis. Opioids also decrease cortisol levels, which results in an increase in fatigue (Benyamin et al., 2008).

Risk vs. Benefit

The following chart shows the authors' interpretation of the literature on the relative effectiveness and risks of various treatments for pain. It is a surreal truth that the most common treatment for chronic pain is the least effective and the most risky.

Efficacy (highest to lowest)	Risk (highest to lowest)
Behavioral treatment	Opioids
Exercise	NSAIDs
Physical therapy	Acetaminophen
Yoga	Antidepressants
Acupuncture	Exercise
Antidepressants	
Anticonvulsants	
NSAIDs	
Acetaminophen	
Opioids	Behavioral tx, exercise, PT, Yoga, Acupuncture have NO risk

Key Points from the Illusion of Opioids

- Opioids are **not very effective** pain relievers.

- Those who take opioids for acute pain experience **many side effects**, and there are even more in those who take these medications for chronic pain.

- Understanding **opioid hyperalgesia** helps us realize that many with chronic pain who start on opioids will have a challenging time ever coming off them and will believe that the opioids are helping (because the pain gets so much worse when they try to go off the medication), when in fact, the opioids may be making the pain—and quality of life—much worse.

- The side effect of **addiction** has affected millions in our country, destroying lives and families. Tens of thousands of individuals die each year from these medications, leaving family members and loved ones to grieve their loss.

Chapter 5

Behavioral Assessment

> *"You must take the first step. The first steps will take some effort, maybe pain.*
> *But after that, everything that has to be done is real-life movement."*
>
> —Ben Stein

It's critically important to do a thorough and careful assessment of a client with chronic pain. It would be a huge mistake to launch into a course of treatment without first knowing everything you can about the person's pain experience.

You will be much more focused in your work with people in chronic pain when you have a solid grasp of their situation and concerns. While professionals may approach this in many different ways, following are some of the important elements of a clinical assessment process.

READINESS FOR CHANGE

One of the first things to assess is the person's readiness for change. Prochaska and DiClemente pioneered the Stages of Change Model in the 1980s, and it's been widely used ever since (Prochaska et al., 2007). It's important to get specific and detailed about what changes the person wants to make. While most people want to reduce their level of pain, it's necessary to get more in depth information about what they have thought about doing that might help. This can give you a idea of what ideas someone has come up with and how practical and realistic those ideas might be. The more someone has thought about what they might do to change, the closer they are to actually changing.

People seek help from professionals for any number of reasons; to get family members off their backs, to satisfy their physicians, to go through the motions to obtain disability status, or to get a prescription. There are also many people who go to a clinician with the hope that they may *finally* get some relief from their chronic pain.

> You may assume that people come to see you because they want you to help them make important changes. Sometimes, that's the case; often it's not.

Motivational Interviewing (MI) can be a useful approach to help people move through the earlier stages toward the action phase. MI is an approach that supports people as they resolve their ambivalence about change. As many of us know from personal experience, change is hard and we often struggle with ambivalence on our way to changing. MI is collaborative and goal-oriented and can help people in chronic pain move through pre-contemplation and contemplation to action.

43

As you look at the following image, consider at what stage of change your client may be. Keep in mind that although the goal is to move toward greater commitment to change, this doesn't always happen in a linear fashion.

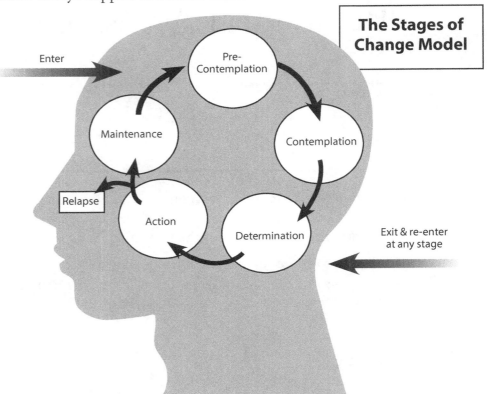

The Stages of Change Model

Enter

Pre-Contemplation

Maintenance

Contemplation

Relapse

Action

Determination

Exit & re-enter at any stage

Let's take a look at the stages in more detail. **Pre-contemplation** is the stage in which people aren't even considering making changes. They may not be resisting change; it's often something that hasn't occurred to them yet. The person with chronic pain may feel hopeless and believe there's nothing that will help; they may not realize that there are tools for reducing pain, even if the medical community can't "fix" the pain.

If you are wondering where to start with someone at this stage, you've got several options. You can open a conversation about change without pushing action. You may want to acknowledge the person's lack of readiness to change, which can make them feel understood and heard. You may also consider helping the person look at their current situation, which may help them start thinking about the possibility of changing. You can also leave the door open for further conversations about change at a later point.

One possible intervention is to help the person shift from an external to an internal locus of control. Empowering someone in that way can have a powerful impact, creating energy and optimism for them to move to the next stage of change.

The **contemplation** stage is often where you'll see people grapple with ambivalence. People may argue with themselves and look at both the costs and the benefits of changing. Change doesn't appear imminent when someone is in the contemplation stage. The person with chronic pain may briefly consider changing but think, "There's nothing that can be done anyway. After all, medical professionals haven't been able to help, so what could I possibly do to improve my pain?"

At this stage, you may address the person's ambivalence and express understanding of their internal conflict. Sometimes, people don't even realize their own ambivalence and can gain more clarity by talking about it. As many of us know (from personal experience!), we don't usually respond well when someone tries to talk us into changing. It's more helpful to acknowledge ambivalence and voice that the decision to change remains that of the person in chronic pain.

Preparation is the stage in which a person is planning to make changes in the near future, perhaps within the next month. They may have made some attempts to change already, and change is something they are looking at in more serious and thoughtful ways. At this point, people with chronic pain have usually already educated themselves about it and know that there are things they can do that may bring relief.

In the preparation phase, you can encourage people to line up social support, try small changes to build success, and identify next steps. Clinicians need to be careful not to take ownership of the change process; rather, they should let this be the client's own journey. This allows clients to own their own success and not attribute all change to their professional team.

The **action** stage involves actually practicing change and implementing new behaviors. Developing new habits takes time, so this stage should last long enough to help the client feel confident in some of the changes they are making. For example, someone with chronic pain may finally start walking around the block, which for them is a breakthrough. We want the person with pain to make the new behavior a habit, not a one-time fluke.

As professionals, we provide tools to help people overcome obstacles, educate them about behavior change, focus on social support, and build confidence. The action phase is when people in pain need lots of practice to create patterns of new behavior.

Maintenance is the phase in which people solidify the new habits and patterns they've developed. This is when they consolidate the gains they've made and feel confident that the changes will be long lasting. The person with chronic pain has a regular activity program or a more active social life. Maybe they are more engaged with family or serving as a volunteer in the community. Your role in the maintenance stage is to help the person build a follow-up plan, have a clear internal locus of control, and identify signs of impending relapse or a slip into old behaviors and patterns.

The **relapse** stage occurs when someone has slipped out of the change, changing habits previously established. Maybe the person with chronic pain has stopped exercising, is withdrawing socially, or is no longer proactive in their own care.

Professionals can help the person identify what may have triggered the decline and help them develop stronger coping skills that are tailored to them. It could be that the client had an illness, which led to a break in their ability to be physically active. Sometimes even a short illness is enough to impact a habit that had been fairly well established. We can help people anticipate things that contribute to relapse and give them tools to prevent it from happening again.

Following is an exercise to share with your clients to help them assess their readiness for change.

My Own Readiness to Change

As you think about readiness for change, it will be helpful for you to figure out where you are in the process. Take a moment to review the following stages of change and select the one that best matches your current thinking and actions.

_____ *(Pre-contemplation)* I haven't really decided to change, and I'm not sure that I need to. I don't know that anything can be done for my chronic pain anyway. Sometimes, I feel pretty hopeless.

_____ *(Contemplation)* I've thought about getting some help for my chronic pain at some point. I don't know that I'm ready right now, but I've considered it.

_____ *(Preparation)* There was a time when I went to a therapist a few times because my doctor suggested it. It helped a bit. I'm thinking about going to see someone again but haven't had time to do it yet. I did get the name of someone who works with chronic pain and may give her a call in the next few weeks.

_____ *(Action)* I've been going through a workbook, and I've seen a therapist a couple of times. I'm trying to be a little more active when I'm having a good day. My family has noticed some changes that I'm working on.

_____ *(Maintenance)* For almost a year, I've been trying to keep up with the changes I've been making. I am not using any pain pills, I'm much more involved with my family, and I'm a lot more productive at work.

_____ *(Relapse)* I was doing pretty well, but then I had an injury and things slid backwards. I got frustrated, and it seemed like I was back at the beginning. It was discouraging, and I didn't cope very well.

Once you've completed this worksheet, you can think about what you might do to move toward the next phase.

If you're in the **pre-contemplation stage**, you can consider your reasons to change. You can weigh the costs and benefits of changing and not changing. Moving to the next stage is totally your decision, and you're much more likely to move ahead if you own that decision and don't feel pressured to make it.

If you fall into the **contemplation stage**, it's important for you to control your own decisions about change and carefully consider the pros and cons of change.

You can do some research and exploring on your own and give some thought to moving to the preparation stage.

If you're in the **preparation stage**, you've decided to make some changes. You can start practicing minor changes and "test the waters" to see how change might feel. Look for opportunities to make small changes and build social support.

Once you're in the **action stage**, you are making some changes, but it's still pretty new. Work to establish new habits and make note of the improvements you're making. Track your progress.

If you're in the **maintenance stage**, you're probably trying to avoid the relapse stage, so you'll want to keep doing what has been helpful. It will be important to work to firmly establish your new habits and changes. Note your improvement and continue to look for ways you can feel even better and stronger. Write down your ideas—it may help you stay on track.

Once you have a **relapse** (which is actually quite common), you can reflect on what might have triggered it. Were you depressed, anxious, discouraged, or frustrated? Did you have an episode of pain and fall into catastrophic thinking? This is a good time to lean on your support system and your treating professionals. Look back *and* look forward. Try to figure out what led to the relapse (look back), and do some things that will get you going in a better direction (look forward).

EVALUATING PAIN

It's essential for behavioral health professionals to work closely with medical providers to properly evaluate someone's pain. A thorough medical workup is a necessity. The medical team can assess the physical aspects of pain and help establish a treatment plan. It's important to have the person with chronic pain sign releases for medical and behavioral health providers to communicate about their care, as collaboration greatly improves outcomes.

Materson (1990) identified 12 elements of pain that should be evaluated as part of a pain assessment. They are:

1. Date of pain onset
2. Circumstances of pain onset
3. Speed of the appearance of the pain
4. Elements that modulate pain
5. Behaviors and attitudes changed by pain
6. Location and intensity of pain
7. History of diagnosis
8. History of treatment
9. History of medications used
10. Other medical history
11. Substance abuse (e.g., alcohol, nicotine, other drugs)
12. Psychological aspects

ASSESSING FOR MENTAL HEALTH AND SUBSTANCE USE ISSUES

Evaluating for possible mental health and substance use issues is a standard part of a pain assessment. As we emphasize throughout this workbook, there is a significant correlation between chronic pain and mental health.

A thorough assessment includes screening for depression, anxiety, and substance use concerns. There are a myriad of screening tools and instruments to identify any possible mental health concerns. A careful assessment of substance use (historical, current, and family history) is essential. This is all part of the evaluation and is the foundation of treatment.

PAIN INTERVIEW

Using a structured pain interview provides consistency and ensures that all of the major areas are being addressed. Otis (2007) has developed a solid interview format that can add structure and documentation to the assessment process.

Following is a worksheet that gives structure to an initial pain interview. You can use this template as you assess people.

Pain Interview

Name _____

Age _____

Evaluation date _____

Completed by _____

Pain Location

Primary pain site _____

Secondary pain site _____

Details of Injury/Onset

_____

_____

Date of Injury/Onset

Primary pain site _____

Secondary pain site _____

Descriptors (e.g., burning, electric, sharp)

_____

_____

Pain Rating (Scale: 0 = No pain; 10 = Worst pain imaginable)

Current _____

Within the past 2 weeks: average _____; worst _____; least _____; intermittent _____; constant _____

Pain Medications and Effectiveness

_____

_____

Previous Treatments (What things have you tried?)

Physical therapy _____

Chiropractic _____

Surgery _____

Psychology _____

Other _____

Temporal Cycles (Have you noticed any patterns to the pain?)

_____

_____

Pain Triggers (What makes your pain increase?)

_____

_____

Pain Reducers (What makes your pain decrease?)

_____

_____

Coping Strategies (How do you cope with pain?)

_____

_____

Litigation Pending?

_____

_____

Personal Goals (What are your goals for treatment?)

_____

_____

Psychosocial History

Childhood (Where did you grow up? With whom did you live?)

_____

_____

Education

_____

_____

Past/Present Occupation

_____

_____

Marital/Family Relationship

_____

_____

Living Situation (Where do you live? With whom? How do they respond to you when you're in pain?)

_____

_____

Recreational Activities

_____

_____

Typical Day (Describe a typical day for you)

_____

_____

Impact of Pain (How has pain impacted your life?)

_____

_____

Substance Use

Past and Present Alcohol and/or Tobacco Use

_____

_____

Past and Present Recreational Drug Use

_____

_____

Affective Status

Prominent Mood Disorders (Have you noticed any changes in your mood? Have you been feeling depressed? Have you experienced any anxiety?)

_____

_____

Past or Present Participation in Individual or Group Therapy

_____

_____

Past or Present Psychiatric Hospitalizations

_____

_____

Psychopharmacological Medications

_____

_____

Developed by John D. Otis, 2007. Reprinted with permission.

THE FIVE E'S OF A PAIN INTERVIEW

Those of you who like simple strategies to remember things might use the "**Five Es of a Pain Interview**." Inspired by MI, this approach makes it more likely that a strong assessment will be the first step toward change.

The first *E* is for **empathy**. It's critical to ask person-centered and open-ended questions. People in chronic pain often feel misunderstood when they come to see yet another professional. They may fear being seen as pill-seekers or fakers.

> Expressing genuine empathy will go a long way toward making clients feel comfortable and understood.

Expressing genuine empathy will go a long way toward making clients feel comfortable and understood.

Our next *E* stands for **evaluate**. That seems obvious, since we're talking about an evaluation, but here, it means something more. During the evaluation, we emphasize making a careful and accurate diagnosis. Clinicians need to be up to date on current diagnostic guidelines as contained in the *DSM-5*® (APA, 2013). We want to determine just what mental health or substance use conditions may be factors in the person's experience.

The third *E* is for **educate**. We are educating people on the disadvantages of the status quo and highlighting the benefits of change. This education piece has a much greater impact when we can work with the person's own ideas, not imposing our ideas and values.

The next *E* stands for **encourage**. Some of the people with whom we're working are short on optimism and long on discouragement. We want to show them that change is possible, even for those with pain that has lasted a long time and seems overwhelming. The goal here is to show our clients that change is possible and could be transformative for them.

The final *E* is the word **engage**. In this portion of the pain interview, we want to engage and join with the person by supporting their intention to change. Even people who are discouraged and pessimistic about the likelihood of living without pain have at least a shred of hope and optimism, or they wouldn't be seeing a professional for help. We want to capitalize and build on that hope.

SELF-REPORT MEASURES

There are several self-report measures that you can use to better understand your client's pain experience. You can rely on these measures to gain a fuller picture of the person's current situation.

Short Form McGill Pain Questionnaire (SF-MPQ)

This is a well-respected measure that covers sensory (11 items) and affective (4 items) aspects of pain. This instrument is reliable, valid, and stable. It's widely used and helpful when doing an assessment. It doesn't take long to fill out and score, making it useful in a wide range of settings.

West Haven-Yale Multidimensional Pain Inventory (WHYMPI)

The WHYMPI offers a comprehensive assessment of functioning. It's a 52-item self-report tool broken into three parts, and it takes about 20 minutes to administer. You'll find the inventory in the next pages.

Part I touches on perceived interference of pain, support or concern from spouse or significant other, pain severity, perceived life control, and affective distress. Part II looks at the person's perceptions of the degree to which spouses or significant others display solicitous, distracting, or negative responses to their pain behaviors and complaints. Part III assesses the person's report of the frequency with which they engage in four categories of common everyday activities.

Numeric Pain Rating Scale

This is probably the simplest tool for understanding a person's recent pain experience. It's quick and straightforward. It uses a range of 0 (no pain at all) to 10 (worst pain imaginable) to rate pain. Ask the person to rate their average, worst, and least pain over the past week. Keep in mind that the numeric pain rating only measures the sensory aspect of pain and does not measure the distress caused by the pain.

There are many different pain scales that help people articulate their level of pain. Take a look at the worksheet to see how a pain scale can be used as part of an assessment. This pain scale is effective because it uses numbers, colors, words, and faces to help people identify their pain level. You can have your client fill it out as often as is useful, it's located on page 60.

Multidimensional Pain Inventory

Before you begin, please answer 2 pre-evaluation questions below:

1. Some of the questions in this questionnaire refer to your "significant other". A significant other is a person with whom you feel closest. This includes anyone that you relate to on a regular or frequent basis. It is very important that you identify someone as your "significant other". Please indicate below who your significant other is (check one):

☐ Spouse ☐ Partner/Companion ☐ Housemate/Roomate ☐ Friend ☐ Neighbor

☐ Parent/Child/Other relative ☐ Other (please describe):

2. Do you currently live with this person? ☐ Yes ☐ No

When you answer questions in the following pages about "your significant other", always respond in reference to the specific person you just indicated above.

A. In the following 20 questions, you will be asked to describe your pain and how it affects your life. Under each question is a scale to record your answer. Read each question carefully and then circle a number on the scale under that question to indicate how that specific question applies to you.

1. Rate the level of your pain at the present moment.

       0   1   2   3   4   5   6
   No pain   Very intense pain

2. In general, how much does your pain problem interfere with your day to day activities?

       0   1   2   3   4   5   6
   No intereference   Extreme interference

3. Since the time you developed a pain problem, how much has your pain changed your ability to work?

       0   1   2   3   4   5   6
   No change   Extreme change

   ____Check here, if you have retired for reasons other than your pain problem.

4. How much has your pain changed the amount of satisfaction or enjoyment you get from participating in social and recreational activities?

       0   1   2   3   4   5   6
   No change   Extreme change

5. How supportive or helpful is your spouse (significant other) to you in relation to your pain?

       0   1   2   3   4   5   6
   Not at all supportive   Extremely supportive

6. Rate your overall mood during the past week.

       0   1   2   3   4   5   6
   Extremely low mood   Extremely high mood

7. On the average, how severe has your pain been during the last week?

       0   1   2   3   4   5   6
   Not at all severe   Extremely severe

8. How much has your pain changed your ability to participate in recreational and other social activities?

       0   1   2   3   4   5   6

No change   Extreme change

9. How much has your pain changed the amount of satisfaction you get from family-related activities?

       0   1   2   3   4   5   6

No change   Extreme change

10. How worried is your spouse (significant other) about you in relation to your pain problem?

       0   1   2   3   4   5   6

Not at all worried   Extremely worried

11. During the past week, how much control do you feel that you have had over your life?

       0   1   2   3   4   5   6

Not at all in control   Extremely in control

12. How much suffering do you experience because of your pain?

       0   1   2   3   4   5   6

No suffering   Extreme suffering

13. How much has your pain changed your marriage and other family relationships?

       0   1   2   3   4   5   6

No change   Extreme change

14. How much has your pain changed the amount of satisfaction or enjoyment you get from work?

       0   1   2   3   4   5   6

No change   Extreme change

_____Check here, if you are not presently working.

15. How attentive is your spouse (significant other) to your pain problem?

       0   1   2   3   4   5   6

Not at all attentive   Extremely attentive

16. During the past week, how much do you feel that you've been able to deal with your problems?

       0   1   2   3   4   5   6

Not at all   Extremely well

17. How much has your pain changed your ability to do household chores?

       0   1   2   3   4   5   6

No change   Extreme change

18. During the past week, how irritable have you been?

       0   1   2   3   4   5   6

Not at all irritable   Extremely irritable

19. How much has your pain changed your friendships with people other than your family?

       0   1   2   3   4   5   6

No change   Extreme change

20. During the past week, how tense or anxious have you been?

       0   1   2   3   4   5   6

Not at all tense or anxious   Extremely tense or anxious

B. In this section, we are interested in knowing how your significant other (this refers to the person you indicated in the first section) responds to you when he or she knows that you are in pain. On the scale listed below each question, **circle a number** to indicate how often your significant other generally responds to you in that particular way when you are in pain.

1. Ignores me.

    0   1   2   3   4   5   6
    Never   Very often

2. Asks me what he/she can do to help.

    0   1   2   3   4   5   6
    Never   Very often

3. Reads to me.

    0   1   2   3   4   5   6
    Never   Very often

4. Expresses irritation at me.

    0   1   2   3   4   5   6
    Never   Very often

5. Takes over my jobs or duties.

    0   1   2   3   4   5   6
    Never   Very often

6. Talks to me about something else to take my mind off the pain.

    0   1   2   3   4   5   6
    Never   Very often

7. Expresses frustration at me.

    0   1   2   3   4   5   6
    Never   Very often

8. Tries to get me to rest.

    0   1   2   3   4   5   6
    Never   Very often

9. Tries to involve me in some activity.

    0   1   2   3   4   5   6
    Never   Very often

10. Expresses anger at me.

    0   1   2   3   4   5   6
    Never   Very often

11. Gets me some pain medications.

    0   1   2   3   4   5   6
    Never   Very often

12. Encourages me to work on a hobby.

    0   1   2   3   4   5   6
    Never   Very often

13. Gets me something to eat or drink.

    0   1   2   3   4   5   6

Never   Very often

14. Turns on the T.V. to take my mind off my pain.

    0   1   2   3   4   5   6

Never   Very often

C. Listed below are 18 common daily activities. Please indicate <u>how often</u> you do each of these activities by <u>circling</u> a number on the scale listed below each activity. Please complete <u>all</u> 18 questions.

1. Wash dishes.

    0   1   2   3   4   5   6

Never   Very often

2. Mow the lawn.

    0   1   2   3   4   5   6

Never   Very often

3. Go out to eat.

    0   1   2   3   4   5   6

Never   Very often

4. Play cards or other games.

    0   1   2   3   4   5   6

Never   Very often

5. Go grocery shopping.

    0   1   2   3   4   5   6

Never   Very often

6. Work in the garden.

    0   1   2   3   4   5   6

Never   Very often

7. Go to a movie.

    0   1   2   3   4   5   6

Never   Very often

8. Visit friends.

    0   1   2   3   4   5   6

Never   Very often

9. Help with the house cleaning.

    0   1   2   3   4   5   6

Never   Very often

10. Work on the car.

    0   1   2   3   4   5   6

Never   Very often

11. Take a ride in a car.

0	1	2	3	4	5	6
Never						Very often

12. Visit relatives.

0	1	2	3	4	5	6
Never						Very often

13. Prepare a meal.

0	1	2	3	4	5	6
Never						Very often

14. Wash the car.

0	1	2	3	4	5	6
Never						Very often

15. Take a trip.

0	1	2	3	4	5	6
Never						Very often

16. Go to a park or beach.

0	1	2	3	4	5	6
Never						Very often

17. Do a load of laundry.

0	1	2	3	4	5	6
Never						Very often

18. Work on a needed house repair.

0	1	2	3	4	5	6
Never						Very often

Numeric Pain Rating Scale

Take a look at this pain rating scale as you consider how your pain has been for the past week.

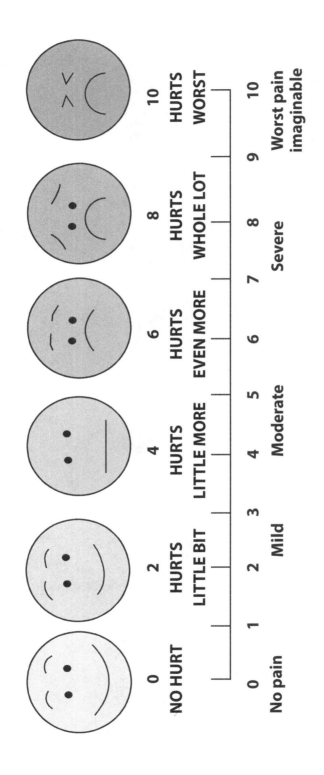

	NO HURT	HURTS LITTLE BIT	HURTS LITTLE MORE	HURTS EVEN MORE	HURTS WHOLE LOT	HURTS WORST
	0	2	4	6	8	10

0	1	2	3	4	5	6	7	8	9	10
No pain		Mild		Moderate			Severe			Worst pain imaginable

Over the past week, what was your average pain level? _____

Over the past week, what was your worst pain level? _____

Over the past week, what was your best pain level? _____

PAIN CATASTROPHIZING SCALE

Many people with chronic pain catastrophize their pain. They imagine the worst possible thing that could happen. They can quickly become overwhelmed and feel helpless and hopeless. Because pain catastrophizing has such a negative impact on the pain experience, it's important to include this as part of the assessment.

The Pain Catastrophizing Scale (PCS) is a well-designed instrument that gives a clear picture of a person's tendency to catastrophize. The subscales include rumination, magnification, and helplessness. It has 13 items and is quick to administer. Scores range from one to four for each item. A score higher than 30 indicates that the person is likely to be a "pain catastrophizer."

People who score about 30 (75th percentile) have much worse outcomes. About 70% are unemployed at one year following their injury, 70% report that they are totally disabled and can't work, and 66% report moderate or severe depression.

You can find this scale on the next pages.

Pain Catastrophizing Scale

Name _____

Age _____

Gender _____

Date _____

Everyone experiences painful situations at some point in their lives. Such experiences may include headaches, tooth pain, or joint or muscle pain. People are often exposed to situations that may cause pain, such as illness, injury, dental procedures, or surgery.

We are interested in the types of thoughts and feelings that you have when you are in pain. Listed below are 13 statements describing different thoughts and feelings that may be associated with pain. Using the following scale, please indicate the degree to which you have these thoughts and feelings when you are experiencing pain.

0 = Not at all

1 = To a slight degree

2 = To a moderate degree

3 = To a great degree

4 = All the time

When I'm in pain . . .

1. _____ I worry all the time about whether the pain will end.

2. _____ I feel I can't go on.

3. _____ It's terrible, and I think it's never going to get any better.

4. _____ It's awful, and I feel that it overwhelms me.

5. _____ I feel I can't stand it anymore.

6. _____ I become afraid that the pain will get worse.

7. _____ I keep thinking of other painful events.

8. _____ I anxiously want the pain to go away.

9. _____ I can't seem to keep it out of my mind.

10. _____ I keep thinking about how much it hurts.

11. _____ I keep thinking about how badly I want the pain to stop.

12. _____ There's nothing I can do to reduce the intensity of the pain.

13. _____ I wonder whether something serious may happen.

_____ TOTAL SCORE

THE IMPACT OF PAIN

Part of the assessment process is determining the impact of pain on someone's life. You need to fully understand this impact so you can better support the person with whom you're working.

We've already established that there is a significant emotional component with chronic pain. In this section, we look at the impact that chronic pain has on people's activities and on their thoughts and feelings.

Chronic pain usually limits people's activity level. It hurts to move around, so people assume it's safer or better to be less active. All of this leads to social withdrawal and deconditioning.

Pain also has a significant impact on people's thoughts and feelings. People with chronic pain often become pessimistic and have a pattern of negative thinking. These thoughts and emotions only make the pain experience worse.

Otis (2007) developed a few questions to assess this impact which we've adapted and included on the following pages. Have your clients fill this out, and take a few minutes to go over the responses with them so you can clearly understand the impact of pain on their activities, thoughts, and emotions.

Assessment is the foundation of chronic pain treatment. With a thorough and careful assessment, you'll have a map for moving forward. Without it, treatment is unfocused and aimless. Take all the time you need to be sure you fully understand your client before you shift into treatment.

The Impact of Pain

Impact on Activity Level

1. How does chronic pain affect your ability to engage in social activities or hobbies?

_____

_____

_____

2. How does chronic pain affect your ability to work or function?

_____

_____

_____

3. When you are in pain, what kinds of activities do you usually do?

_____

_____

_____

4. What kind of negative physical or social effects come from limiting your activities?

_____

_____

_____

Impact of Thoughts and Feelings

1. What relationship do you observe between your emotions and pain?

_____

_____

_____

2. How do you feel emotionally on days when you are experiencing a lot of pain?

_____

_____

_____

3. In what ways do anger, frustration, or sadness increase with pain?

_____

_____

_____

4. What kinds of thoughts are associated with those feelings?

_____

_____

_____

Adapted from John D. Otis, 2007

Key Points of Behavioral Assessment

- It is vitally important that you assess a person's **readiness for change**. This allows you to meet your client where they are and help them move closer to behavioral change.

  The **stages of change** include:

    - Pre-contemplation

    - Contemplation

    - Preparation

    - Action

    - Maintenance

    - Relapse

- A structured **pain interview** can be of great help as you complete a thorough and comprehensive assessment.

- The **5 E's** of a pain interview can help frame your approach to someone with chronic pain. The 5 E's are:

    - Empathy

    - Evaluation

    - Education

    - Encouragement

    - Engagement

- **Self-report measures** are a useful part of the assessment process. Well-supported measures include:

    - Short Form McGill Pain Questionnaire (SF-MPQ)

    - West Haven-Yale Multidimensional Pain Inventory (WHYMPI)

    - Numeric Pain Rating Scale

    - Pain Catastrophizing Scale (PCS)

- The **impact of pain** on activities and on thoughts and feelings can be determined by using a simple questionnaire that includes four questions for each of those domains.

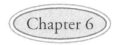

Chapter 6

Goal Setting and Special Populations

> *"Men who have pierced ears are better prepared for marriage –*
> *they've experienced pain and bought jewelry."*
>
> —*Rita Rudner*

As we move out of the assessment phase and into the goal-setting process, remember the robust value of the therapeutic relationship. Outcome studies consistently reinforce the importance of the relationship between therapist and client.

Many "nonspecific factors" have a significant impact on people's progress in treatment. These include empathy, clinician support, and the ability to motivate, understand, and personalize treatment preferences and expectations, which are vital in facilitating change. We also have an abundance of data that show that a positive client-clinician relationship reduces pain and disability. A solid program of behavioral treatment with a skilled professional allows clients to use fewer medications and report less pain. This is reflected in the 2016 guidelines on the treatment of chronic pain published by the CDC. The CDC guidelines favor behavioral treatment rather than continued reliance on opioids.

> The 2016 CDC guidelines for the treatment of chronic pain favor behavioral treatment rather than continued reliance on opioids.

GOAL SETTING

Once you've completed a thorough assessment of someone with chronic pain, it's time to develop goals. You will do this in collaboration with the person so you can be sure that you aren't just working on *your* goals for them but are connecting with what is important to them. As you work on this together, you are learning a tremendous amount about what's important to the individual, and you can help weave their values together with their goals.

Helping people develop behavioral goals can be a powerful intervention in itself. The language around behavioral goals tends to be action-oriented and proactive rather than passive and reactive. People feel an internal locus of control rather than an external locus of control with behavioral goals. This can build a sense of empowerment and optimism.

Otis (2007) suggests three types of therapeutic goals: overall treatment goals, weekly behavioral goals, and homework goals. **Overall treatment goals** include realistic and short-term goals that can be achieved during the weeks or months of treatment, as opposed to long-term goals, which can take months or years to complete. These are specific rather than vague and can be adjusted over time as the person's needs change. You'll want to help your clients develop new goals to shoot for as they accomplish their earlier goals.

Weekly behavioral goals are small goals that can be accomplished between sessions. These can be set up in small increments to build successes. For example, someone whose goal is to start a walking program can begin with a goal of walking twice a week for 10 minutes, gradually increasing frequency and duration as appropriate.

Homework goals are related to what is discussed during a session. These goals are linked to the content of the session with an eye toward practicing new skills. If you have worked on mindfulness tools during a session, a natural goal could be to practice relaxation breathing a certain number of times before the next session.

Be aware of the importance of individualizing goals to be in sync with your clients' values. Not all goals fit for all people. Matching people's values with their goals instead of taking a one-size-fits-all approach will allow you to accomplish several important things. The person will see a reduced negative impact of pain on their daily life, they'll experience improved physical and emotional functioning, they'll increase effective coping skills to manage pain, and they'll report reduced pain intensity.

> Matching people's values with their goals instead of taking a one-size-fits-all approach will allow you to accomplish several important things.

Many people haven't thought much about what their goals are. Perhaps they've had a hard time imagining themselves getting better and have developed pessimism about their chances of improvement. After all, they have probably seen several professionals and haven't gotten "fixed" yet. Talking with your clients about their goals can move them toward a more positive and optimistic view of their future. This conversation shifts their focus from chronic pain to better functioning.

You can present some general goals of treatment to begin a discussion about the person's individual goals. A few general treatment goals may include:

- Reducing pain and the use of pain medication
- Developing tools to cope with pain more effectively
- Improving functioning, both physically and emotionally
- Minimizing the impact of pain on daily life and relationships

You can guide the discussion in ways that help your clients articulate their personal goals. This may be a new way of thinking for them that can help open up some different views of what they might be able to accomplish. Here are some ideas of questions you could ask to help them uncover some personal goals:

- What is one specific thing you'd like to see improvement in over the next weeks and months?
- What would you like to do more of as your pain improves?
- How might your relationships change for the better when your pain is reduced?
- How will your life be better when you can manage your pain differently?

SMART goals is an approach to goal setting that can be incredibly useful as you develop a treatment plan with people. SMART goals are:

- Specific: The person can identify a specific action or event that will occur
- Measurable: The goal should be quantifiable and able to be measured
- Achievable: The goal is realistic and able to be attained
- Relevant: The goal is meaningful to the person
- Time bound: A time frame has been set for when the goal will be reached

It is important to track people's progress toward the goals they have set for themselves. You can help your clients develop accountability by asking about their goals at every session.

> You have probably heard about SMART goals. This approach to goal setting can be incredibly useful as you develop a treatment plan with people.

The following worksheet can be helpful in developing SMART goals.

Worksheet

SMART Goals

SMART goals have several important parts. Think about a goal that you have for yourself. You may have several goals, so you can complete this worksheet for each one of them. As you consider the goal that you have, take some time to work through the following elements of SMART goals.

Specific: Be as specific as possible about your goal. Include as many details as possible. If you want to walk more often, how will you make that happen? Who will you walk with? Where will you walk? When will you do this? Jot down some specific ideas about reaching a goal that you have.

_____

_____

_____

_____

Measurable: Think about how you will measure what you're doing. How will you quantify and track your progress? If your goal is to walk more, how often do you want to walk? How far do you plan to go? How quickly or slowly do you want to walk? Write down how you might measure your progress.

_____

_____

_____

_____

Achievable: Take some time to explore the likelihood that your goal can be achieved. Try to set a goal that you have a good chance of reaching. It's essential to build some successes as you try to make these kinds of changes. Using our walking example, if you've never walked much at all, it would be unreasonable and probably not achievable to have a goal of walking several miles at first or running in a 5K race. What makes your goal achievable?

_____

_____

_____

_____

Relevant: Set a goal that is meaningful to you. You are much more likely to see success if you set a goal that is important to you. Just because a goal seems like a good idea in general doesn't mean that it's personally meaningful to you. What about your goal makes it meaningful to you?

_____

_____

_____

_____

Time bound: Now give some thought to a time frame for your goal. When might you start? When do you think you'll complete this goal?

_____

_____

_____

_____

You can use this same process for any goal you have for any area of your life. Using the SMART goal format can help you be much more successful in achieving any goals you set for yourself.

SPECIAL POPULATIONS

There is a great deal of diversity among people with chronic pain. If we assume there are about 100 million people in the United States with chronic pain, it's a safe bet that they are of all genders, ages, ethnicities, socioeconomic statuses, sexual orientations, and backgrounds. We need to pay careful attention to the varied experiences of a few groups of people with chronic pain so we can tailor treatment to their specific needs.

CHILDREN AND PAIN

Children experience pain even from birth. In years past, it was assumed that infants didn't experience pain, which led to minimal use of medications or anesthesia. We now know that babies do feel pain, and the consequences of that pain exist even after the pain has stopped. Newborns who have frequent blood samples taken begin to anticipate the pain, as evidenced by their reactions to having their heels disinfected prior to the needle stick.

Further evidence of the lasting impact of pain in infancy comes from what we see in babies who experience many painful procedures after birth. They have more psychological, behavioral, emotional, and learning challenges in childhood. These personality-related and behavioral consequences last well into their childhood and teen years.

Recurrent pain is a shockingly common condition in children; it's estimated that about 30% of children have chronic pain, which is comparable to the rates in adults. Marchand (2012) describes the features of recurrent pain in childhood as follows:

- Many painful episodes can occur with no specific pattern over a time from months to years.
- Pain during these episodes may start suddenly and severely or slowly and gradually.
- The pain may last from a few minutes to a few days, most commonly two to three hours.
- Pain can come on any time during waking hours, but it doesn't usually awaken the child.
- Predicting the intensity, duration, or timing of the next episode is impossible.
- There isn't a diagnosed condition that clearly explains the pain.
- There may be a number of triggers, but none of them predictably cause pain every time.
- The pain seems to be related to environmental and emotional factors.
- More girls than boys experience recurrent pain in childhood.

Headaches are the most common form of recurrent pain in children, with a 20% incidence. That incidence tends to increase with age. A good portion of children with headaches also have anxiety, worry, hypersensitivity, and obsessive-compulsive disorder–type traits. In many of these cases, one of the parents had similar issues in childhood.

Abdominal pain is the next most common type of recurrent pain in children, with a 10% to 18% incidence and the highest occurrence being between ages eight and ten years. Lavigne and colleagues (1986) found that several features correlate with abdominal pain: somatization, poor adaptation to stress, depressive tendencies, family history, insecurity, fear of failure or danger, desire for success, and imitation. Children with abdominal pain often live in families where illness and pain are a large part of family life. In such instances, the question of nature versus nurture hasn't been settled.

> A good portion of children with headaches also have anxiety, worry, hypersensitivity, and obsessive-compulsive disorder–type traits. In many of these cases, one of the parents had similar issues in childhood.

Limb pain, also called *growing pains*, typically affects children who are eight to twelve years old. Incidence rates are between 4% and 15%. There is no clear physical cause, and there isn't a tremendous amount of growth between ages eight and twelve. This phenomenon is often linked to emotions and sometimes to family stress, but research is scant.

Central sensitization appears to be a major component in most types of pediatric pain. This means that behavioral treatment will have a much greater impact than other modalities on pain reduction.

Some of the treatment options for children are similar to those for adults. Relaxation and mindfulness techniques can be effective. Exposure therapy (a cognitive-behavioral foundational approach) can ease reactivity to pain and modify cognitive distortions. Other cognitive approaches show promise, such as imagery and thought substitution. Expressive and creative outlets can provide fun, pleasure, and distraction from pain. Hypnosis is also a powerful intervention that may relieve chronic pain in children.

Family dynamics certainly contribute to stress in children, and stress exacerbates pain. High levels of parental anxiety around a child's pain end up worsening the pain, as the children's own fears are magnified. Parents can catastrophize when their children are in pain, making the emotional consequences more problematic for both parents and children. This makes a compelling case for family therapy as an effective intervention. Family-focused strategies can promote healthy responses to a child's chronic pain for both the child and the entire family.

PAIN IN THE ELDERLY

Elderly people are at much greater risk of having chronic pain than younger people. The literature shows that more than 50% of the elderly experience chronic pain. This is due, in part, to the increased number of medical and degenerative conditions with which they live. From chronic diseases to musculoskeletal issues, there are myriad reasons for increased chronic pain in older people.

Additional relevant (non-physical) contributors to geriatric chronic pain include mobility problems, more dependence on others, losses, financial strain, social withdrawal, and isolation. Depression often exists in the elderly and adds to their pain experience. Elders who are depressed have more pain, and those who have chronic pain are three times more likely to develop depression. This emphasizes the need to consider both emotional and physical conditions when treating older people with pain.

As with other age groups with chronic pain, treatment suggestions include increasing physical activity. Added benefits come when this can be blended with social interaction, such as working out in a gym around other people or walking with friends.

Occupational and physical therapy can be powerful interventions as well. Mindfulness activities are helpful, as are spiritual activities based on the individual's values.

PAIN AND GENDER

There are distinct differences in how men and women experience chronic pain. Many of these are related to biological factors and hormonal differences. We know that women tend to have higher ACE scores than men do. This link between childhood trauma and later incidence of chronic pain is part of the reason women have a higher incidence of fibromyalgia and other pain conditions.

Other considerations include psychological, emotional, and social contrasts between men and women. Marchand (2012) describes gender issues related to anxiety, depression, emotional responses, and cognitive factors.

Anxiety is connected to hypervigilance and catastrophizing. High levels of anxiety increase a person's perception of pain. Interestingly, the more anxiety a male has, the greater the perception of pain he will have. This seems to be unique to men. Men also feel more anxiety about pain than women do.

Depression not only increases the risk of chronic pain but also raises the number of complaints of clinical pain. Chronic pain leads to more episodes of depression. Between 30% and 65% of people with chronic pain have depression. Women with depression and chronic pain have increased bodily awareness.

Emotional responses also differ between men and women. Marchand's research shows that women experience more frustration, and men are more anxious. All negative emotions are connected with greater intensity of and sensitivity to pain.

Cognitive factors influence how men and women experience pain. Women use emotional and social supports to deal with pain, whereas men us active, problem-solving techniques. One of the theories around this is that because women perceive more pain than men, they've developed different ways of dealing with it.

Marchand (2012) reports that the literature shows the following:

- Women and men react differently to emotional stimuli
- Women react more to negative stimuli
- Women have more negative emotions related to pain

Key Points of Goal Setting and Special Populations

- **Goal setting** is a collaborative process between you and your client. Goals need to fit with the values of the client and be goals that you can support.

- Goals may be **overall goals**, **weekly goals**, **or homework-related goals**.

- **SMART goals** are those that are specific, measurable, achievable, realistic, and time bound.

- **Children** have chronic pain at the same rate as adults. Research is scant, though there is significant impact on school performance, family functioning, and emotions.

- **The elderly** are at much greater risk of developing chronic pain, with about 50% prevalence. Pain comes with many other complicating factors such as loss, isolation, mobility problems, dependence, and financial strain.

- **Women** experience some unique issues related to pain. They tend to have a higher incidence of pain conditions. They often report greater depression and frustration.

Chapter 7

Non-Opioid Medical Treatment Options

> *"High heels are pleasure with pain."*
> —*Christian Louboutin*

Pain is a complicated and complex experience that affects the physical, psychological, and spiritual aspects of a person's life. Over time, there have been multiple guidelines and ideas about how to best treat chronic pain. Unfortunately, most of these consider opioid medications as the default treatment for chronic pain.

> The CDC guidelines recommend behavioral interventions prior to medications, and are clear that most cases of chronic pain should not be treated with opioid medications.

In 2016, the CDC published the current standard for treatment of chronic pain. This is the first guideline that recommends nonopioid treatment as the *preferred* treatment. The CDC guidelines recommend behavioral interventions prior to medications, and are clear that most cases of chronic pain should *not* be treated with opioid medications.

This chapter focuses on nonopioid *medical* treatments for pain, including medications and alternative therapies, in preparation for the following chapters, which focus on the most effective treatment—behavioral therapy.

MEDICATIONS

There are several nonopioid medications that have some effectiveness in the treatment of chronic pain. None provide dramatic relief, and few have an official FDA indication for treatment of chronic pain. All should be used as a part of a comprehensive pain treatment plan, with behavioral treatment as the centerpiece.

Although the combination of **ibuprofen and acetaminophen** is very effective for acute pain, their utility in chronic pain is more limited. These medicines have little or no effect on pain that is caused by central sensitization. They will have some effect in any pain that has a nociceptive component, such as arthritis. Fibromyalgia and chronic headaches have little or no nociceptive input, so these medications are not helpful for individuals with those diagnoses.

Amitriptyline is a very old antidepressant. Low doses may be helpful in many cases of chronic pain regardless of the etiology. Given at bedtime, it causes drowsiness and will help people sleep better. Improved sleep can reduce chronic pain, and this may explain some of amitriptyline's effectiveness. Unfortunately, amitriptyline may cause drowsiness throughout the day as well. It also stimulates the appetite and may cause weight gain, which is not helpful in chronic pain. Many people will not be able to tolerate these side effects. This medicine is effective in central sensitization and neuropathic pain. Amitriptyline is in the class of drugs called **tricyclic antidepressants**, and other medications in this class may be helpful with fewer side effects.

Other **antidepressants** can also be helpful in the treatment of chronic pain. Duloxetine (Cymbalta) and venlafaxine (Effexor) have FDA indications for treatment of pain; however, all antidepressants probably have pain-relieving effects.

Gabapentin (Neurontin) and **pregabalin (Lyrica)** are both effective for neuropathic pain. Pregabalin is a schedule IV controlled substance and likely has some addiction potential. Both of these drugs also may provide some calming effects in those with anxiety.

Muscle relaxers seldom have much benefit in the treatment of chronic pain. However, **baclofen** may be helpful if there is a large component of muscle spasm causing the pain. **Cyclobenzaprine (Flexeril)** may be helpful if given at bedtime in much the same manner as amitriptyline. **Carisoprodol (Soma)** can be addicting and probably has no benefit when used for chronic pain. It may be deadly when taken with opioids for pain, and its use should be avoided.

INVASIVE TREATMENTS

People with pain often want a fast and easy solution. Unfortunately, this is seldom possible. There are a number of invasive procedures that may be helpful if the major cause of the pain is nociceptive or neuropathic. If central sensitization or opioid withdrawal is a major factor, then the procedures are less likely to be helpful.

> There are several invasive procedures that may be helpful if the major cause of the pain is nociceptive or neuropathic. If central sensitization or opioid withdrawal is a major factor, then the procedures are less likely to be helpful.

Back surgery may be helpful if there is a herniated intervertebral disc that is pushing against a nerve and causing neuropathic pain. By relieving the pressure on the sciatic nerve, neuropathic pain can be relieved. A herniated disc causing nerve impingement in the lower back is often called **sciatica**. Sciatica causes pain in the leg, not the back. For this reason, surgery to relieve sciatic nerve pressure will relieve the leg pain (and numbness) but not back pain. Surgery may also be helpful in spinal stenosis and some other back conditions. Often, however, surgery will not completely relieve the pain.

Epidural steroid injections can be helpful for some back conditions, particularly those with neuropathic pain from a herniated disc or spinal stenosis. Not everyone will get pain relief from this procedure, and for those who do, relief is temporary. As with back surgery, epidural steroid injections relieve sciatica pain but likely will not help pain that is felt in the back.

Nerve blocks involve the injection of a numbing medication around the nerve that is damaged and causing neuropathic pain. These are usually used for diagnostic purposes but may provide some temporary pain relief.

Radiofrequency nerve ablation is used to destroy the nerves that carry pain signals from inflamed joints in the back or neck. This procedure destroys nociceptive nerves and therefore is only effective in relieving nociceptive pain. Most cases of chronic back and neck pain are multifactorial, and the nociceptive component is minimal compared with the central sensitization or neuropathic components.

Spinal cord stimulation involves the placement of an electrical stimulator in the back near the spinal column. The goal is to replace the pain transmission along the spinal column with a more pleasant tingling or numbness. This may be effective in those who have failed multiple back surgeries and in others with chronic back pain.

Spinal cord medication infusion may be helpful in some types of treatment-resistant pain. Opioids or muscle relaxers may be infused around the spinal cord to give some benefit without as many systemic side effects as when they are taken orally. There are some systemic effects, however, and tolerance and hyperalgesia may still occur when opioids are used in this fashion.

Joint replacement can be very effective in those with severe arthritis of particular joints. Those with a large central sensitization component and those on chronic opioids prior to surgery often have worse outcomes and continued pain after surgery.

OTHER NONINVASIVE, NON-MEDICATION TREATMENTS

There are a number of other treatments for chronic pain that do not involve an invasive procedure or prescription medication. Exercise, in particular, is very effective for most types of chronic pain. Other treatments, such as yoga, spinal manipulation, acupuncture, and tai chi may be effective. A review article published in *The Mayo Clinic Proceedings* looked at some of these therapies. A summary table follows on page 82. In general, most alternative therapies are safe and may have some benefit, so they are worth trying if your client is interested (Nahin, Boineau, Khalsa, Stussman, & Weber, 2016).

Key Points from Non-Opioid Medical Treatment Options

- Medications and medical treatments are just **not very effective** treatment for chronic pain.

- It is important that the individual with chronic pain **not expect** the medical community to be the answer to their pain.

TABLE 3. Summary of Evidence for Selected Complementary Health Approaches by Type of Pain (Sham or Placebo and/or Attention Controls)[a,b]

Approach	Back pain	Fibromyalgia	OA of knee	Neck pain	Severe headache/migraine
Acupuncture	1 Positive trial, 2 negative	1 Positive trial, 3 negative trials	1 Positive trial, 3 negative	NA	NA
Chondroitin	NA	NA	1 Negative trial	NA	NA
Glucosamine	NA	NA	2 Positive trials, 3 negative trials	NA	NA
Chondroitin and glucosamine	NA	NA	1 Positive trial, 2 negative trials	NA	NA
Massage therapy	1 Positive trial	NA	NA	2 Positive trials	1 Positive trial
MSM	NA	NA	1 Positive trial	NA	NA
Omega-3 fatty acids	NA	NA	NA	NA	1 Negative trial
Relaxation approaches	NA	1 Positive trial, 2 negative	NA	NA	3 Positive trials
SAMe	NA	NA	NA	NA	NA
Spinal manipulation	6 Positive trials, 3 negative	NA	NA	1 Negative trial	1 Positive trial
Osteopathic manipulation	1 Positive trial, 1 negative	NA	NA	NA	NA
Tai chi	NA	2 Positive trials	3 Positive trials	NA	NA
Yoga	1 Positive trial	NA	1 Positive trial	NA	NA

[a]MSM = methylsulfonylmethane; OA = osteoarthritis; NA = no US randomized controlled trials identified; SAMe = S-adenosylmethionine.
[b]Positive trials are those in which the complementary approach provided statistically significant improvements in pain severity or pain-related disability or function compared with the control group. Negative trials are those in which no difference was seen between groups.

(Nahin, Boineau, Khalsa, Stussman, & Weber, 2016) Reprinted with permission.

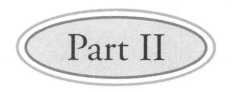

Part II

Behavioral Treatment of Chronic Pain—The Best Answer

> *"Find a place inside where there's joy,*
> *and the joy will burn out the pain."*
> —*Joseph Campbell*

The great majority of people with chronic pain are able to tolerate their pain and will not seek treatment from you or from their physician. For those who do seek help, most commonly they are prescribed medications initially and may undergo one or more procedures meant to alleviate the pain. These may be the two most *ineffective* treatments for chronic pain because they are based on a linear concept of pain, where the nociceptor is triggered by a painful stimulus and the signals are transmitted to the brain, where pain is felt.

Unfortunately chronic pain is much more complicated. Pain is made worse by our emotions, memories, fears, behaviors, social situations, and many other factors. They not only make the pain worse but also adversely affect our ability to cope with it.

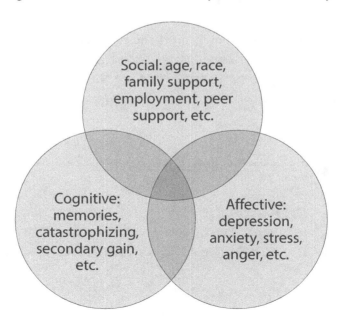

Factors in Chronic Pain

We now know that our brains are not static organs but that they change throughout our lives. These changes generally help us adapt and survive. Although these brain changes are advantageous with acute pain, they are not beneficial with chronic pain. Changes occur in gray matter, white matter, and neural pathways, which lead to central sensitization and the ongoing perception of pain even *without* nociceptive input. Thus, all the medical procedures in the world will not relieve the pain.

Many experts today are saying that we need to embrace a new model of chronic pain as a disease of the central nervous system and not of the musculoskeletal system if we want to improve outcomes for chronic pain treatment (Pelletier et al., 2015). Some pain experts have gone as far as to say that we should change the definition of chronic pain to "pain that does not extinguish its memory trace" (Mansour et al., 2014), highlighting the central nervous system as the central pathology.

The good news is, these brain changes do not have to be permanent. It is possible to reverse these problematic alterations. Science has shown that behavioral treatments can rewire the brain to make it work better again. Medications cannot do this. Medicines may reduce the pain somewhat, but they don't fix the problem. In fact, opioids probably make it worse, as they also cause changes that magnify the pain.

In the past 10 years, there has been an explosion of functional MRI studies that show not only the structure of the brain but also neural pathways and how they work. Many studies have confirmed the physical changes of the brain from pain. Many have also shown that cognitive-behavioral therapy, mindfulness therapy, meditation, and exercise help reverse these changes and heal the brain.

Let's say you have a client who comes in with chronic back pain. He has suffered from his pain for many years. He has had multiple injections and several operations. None of them have helped. Medications have not helped. Do you see the problem? The medical community is treating the wrong thing. Clinicians have been taught that if the pain is in the back, then the problem is in the back. But it is not. The problem is in the brain, which has been changed by the chronic pain. It is a complicated problem, and no neurosurgeon can fix it. But as a clinician, you can! The remaining chapters introduce you to the techniques you will need to change brains and make them better.

> The medical community is treating the wrong thing. Clinicians have been taught that if the pain is in the back, then the problem is in the back. But it is not. The problem is in the brain, which has been changed by the chronic pain.

Chapter 8

Mindfulness for Chronic Pain

> *"It is easier to find men who will volunteer to die,*
> *than to find those who are willing to endure pain with patience."*
> —*Julius Caesar*

Mindfulness practices are proven, effective, and powerful interventions for people with chronic pain. These approaches are easy to learn and can be incorporated into people's lives in ways that bring comfort, relaxation, and decreased pain.

Jon Kabat-Zinn, developer of Mindfulness-Based Stress Reduction, describes mindfulness as "paying attention in a particular way; on purpose, in the present moment, non-judgmentally." Others have simply said that to be mindful you should "be where you are." You can "be where you are" both in place and time—being present in the here and now and not dwelling on the past or future. You can help people notice and fully engage in the present moment without harsh judgment of their thoughts.

The essence of mindfulness is being aware of your thoughts, your surroundings, and your current experience in a way that is observational and reflective, not critical and reactive. By calming your reactivity, you can actually change the way your body and mind respond.

> The essence of mindfulness is being aware of your thoughts, your surroundings, and your current experience in a way that is observational and reflective, not critical and reactive.

Taking a nonjudgmental stance toward yourself is a kinder, gentler approach than being harsh and critical with yourself. We often judge our experiences and situations as good or bad, negative or positive. These automatic, quick assessments prevent us from carefully observing and describing things more fully.

Being aware of your present experience with acceptance brings contentment rather than inner turmoil. When people with chronic pain are able to do this, they are able to observe their pain with much less reactivity.

People with chronic pain who practice mindfulness have less anticipatory pain anxiety. A mindful approach also fosters cognitive change and openness. People often report that they can tolerate pain differently and find it less distressing and unpleasant.

Once a mindful practice is established, people can observe their thoughts more objectively, see more clearly how their beliefs impact their pain, and modify their cognitive distortions more effectively. People who cultivate a mindful approach can calmly evaluate and regulate their initial emotional responses. An example of this could be, "I'm noticing pain in my back, but I probably overdid it when I was working in the yard today. I'll wait and see what happens with it."

This ability to manage reactions has stunning results for people with chronic pain. We know that pain is a stress response. The body (and mind) experience chronic pain in ways that are similar to how they experience chronic stress. Consider the similarities in how our nervous system responds to both stress and pain.

With pain and stress, we experience distressing thoughts, rapid heartbeat, quick and shallow breathing, constricted blood vessels, muscle tightness, with cortisol and inflammatory factors being released into the bloodstream. These experiences are related to the fight, freeze, or flight response. Our **sympathetic nervous system** pumps out adrenaline and other stress hormones when we are in danger. Our bodies are on high alert. This can be adaptive when we are threatened, but in the case of chronic stress and chronic pain, this becomes problematic. A stress response is no longer helpful, since it wears out the body, depletes essential hormones, and exhausts the mind.

The **parasympathetic nervous system** controls heart rate, blood pressure, digestion, relaxation, healing, rest, and a healthy immune system. People with chronic pain often have a stressed

> Pain impacts stress, and stress impacts pain. There is a strong, unavoidable link.

and overworked sympathetic nervous system, which leads to fatigue and additional strain on the body.

Combine chronic stress with chronic pain and you've got a challenging mix. In addition to the stress of physical pain, there's often the added stress of challenging family dynamics, financial concerns, social isolation, decreased activity, and drop in self-worth.

This is where mindfulness shines. Using mindful approaches dials down the fight, freeze, or flight reaction and allows for a calmer assessment of circumstances. The parasympathetic nervous system kicks in and brings us to a more relaxed and peaceful state of being. This not only eases the mind but actually reduces physical pain as well. Mindful approaches directly target these stress reactions, dramatically weakening their impact on our bodies and thoughts.

THE RELAXATION RESPONSE

The **Relaxation Response** was originally developed by Herbert Benson of Harvard Medical School back in the 1970s. This is a profound yet simple way to quiet our bodies' reactivity to stress, including chronic pain. The benefits are both physical and mental. Benson's research clearly showed that practicing the Relaxation Response helps subdue our sympathetic nervous systems, making it harder for our bodies to become reactive to stressors (such as chronic pain). We are less likely to have a fight, freeze, or flight response. This leads us to be less aroused by chronic stress symptoms.

> The Relaxation Response has a couple of priorities: focusing on a repetitive breath, word, action, or phrase and developing a passive attitude toward thoughts that go through our heads.

This approach has a couple of priorities: focusing on a repetitive breath, word, action, or phrase and developing a passive attitude toward thoughts that go through our heads. Having a more passive attitude toward our thoughts leads us to greater acceptance than if we were to fight against those thoughts.

The Relaxation Response has both immediate and long-term benefits. Short-term improvements include what happens as we're practicing our response, which may include lower blood pressure, slower heart rate, calmer breathing, and better blood oxygen levels. Longer-term gains may be an improvement in how the body responds to adrenaline, less anxiety and depression, and a better ability to handle stress. The long-term benefits are experienced even when the person is not currently practicing the Relaxation Response.

BREATHING

We all breathe. It's an automatic behavior necessary for life. Once we stop breathing, we are no longer alive. Why devote our attention to it? Although breathing is essential to life, many of us only breathe well enough to keep ourselves alive but not in a way that brings restoration, healing, and relaxation. In fact, most of us pay very little attention to our breathing unless we're congested, sick, or struggling to breathe for some other reason.

Breathing is a great mindfulness entry point for people with chronic pain. The guidance that we give is simple and easy to learn. People are usually open to trying new breathing techniques and are happily surprised with the immediate results. Once people realize how well breathing techniques work, they're often inspired to do them regularly.

We want people with chronic pain to experience the link between their breathing and their pain. Breathing well brings relief both physically and mentally. There is an element of distraction, since when we focus on our breathing, we're not focusing on our pain. There are also strong physical changes that come when we breathe well.

Here's an experiment to try with someone who has chronic pain. Ask the person to make a tight fist and hold it. Ask them to notice what happens with their breathing. They'll usually report that they are holding their breath or taking shallow and tight breaths. Now ask them to breathe using slow, deep breaths, then to make a fist while continuing to breathe deeply. They will probably report that they weren't able to make a very tight fist while maintaining slow and deep breathing. The breathing actually makes it hard to hold tension and stress.

Let's take a look at an exercise that you can go over with your clients in session. You can also have them take a copy home with them so they can refer to it later.

It can be helpful to do these exercises with your client when you first ask them to try them. This helps ease any self-consciousness on the client's part and provides modeling that will help them learn the techniques well.

You may want to suggest that your clients keep a log of when they practice breathing exercises and what the results were. This helps them keep track of their progress and reinforces the positive benefits that are derived. You can ask people to bring their logs with them to appointments so you can ago over them together and highlight progress and success.

Following the Relaxation Breathing handout is a log that you can share with your clients. Take a look at this with your clients in session so you can explain it and answer any questions about it.

Relaxation Breathing

One of the most important things you can do to help with your pain is to observe your breathing and notice how it affects your physical pain and emotional stress. This is a simple process and can be done anywhere, anytime. You'll notice immediate results, and with frequent practice, you'll be able to develop breathing habits that benefit you in the long term. You'll notice that your breathing will become slower and deeper.

- Start by making yourself comfortable. You can sit in a chair with your feet on the ground. Relax your body as much as you can. Try to shut out distractions—no TV, music, or chaos around you—especially as you're just starting out.

- Breathe in slowly through your nose. Hold it a moment and slowly breathe out. Repeat two or three times. You may already notice that your body relaxes as you do this. Take another couple of breaths in and out of your nose. What do you notice about the temperature of the air when you breathe in and when you breathe out? Is the temperature different when you inhale than when you exhale?

Now we'll focus on deep breathing, sometimes called **diaphragmatic breathing**, since we're focusing on the diaphragm. Most of us move our chest when we breathe while our belly doesn't move. We'll get a much more effective result if we move our belly.

- Put one hand on your chest and one on your belly. Breathe in and out. What part moves more, your chest or your belly?

- Take a few more slow breaths and purposely try to move your belly in and out as you breathe. When you do this, you'll get the full benefit of more air in your lungs, slower breathing, increased oxygen intake, and more energy.

- As you breathe in and out you might imagine yourself breathing out pain and stress while breathing in relaxation.

- Gently bring your focus back as your thoughts wander, which they will. Practice a bit of self-compassion and understand that thoughts may stray and you can gently bring them back.

Practice this several times daily, gradually increasing the time you spend. Like anything else, it takes practice to become comfortable when learning something new.

Breathing Practice Log

As you practice your new breathing exercises, it may help you to use this log to mark your progress. This can support you in developing new habits and assist you as you look at the benefits you're experiencing. Please bring this back when you come in for your appointments so we can talk about how you're doing.

Date and time

_____

Setting (Where I was, what was going on around me)

_____

My pain level (0–10) before I began the breathing practice

_____

My stress level (0–10) before I began

_____

What I practiced

_____

My pain level (0–10) when I was done with the breathing exercise

_____

My stress level (0–10) when I was done

_____

Other thoughts

_____

What I might want to try the next time I do this

_____

IMAGERY

We can help people with chronic pain find relief, both mentally and physically, when we help them use imagery in a meaningful way. People with chronic pain can experience improvement by using positive, healing, peaceful imagery. This is a skill that people can use anytime and anywhere. It can become a useful and portable mindfulness tool to help combat the stress that goes along with chronic pain. As you introduce the concept of imagery, you can go through the following worksheet with your clients.

Worksheet

Imagery

As a person with chronic pain, you can relax your mind and reduce your pain by practicing imagery. This worksheet will guide you as you start to use imagery as a mindfulness tool. Before you start, make sure that you are comfortable and have a few minutes without interruption.

Use your imagination to be as specific as possible as you think about the following questions. Try to get in touch with all of your senses. As you picture a place, imagine how you might enter it (e.g., through a door, on a trail). It may help to close your eyes as you imagine this place.

Setting: Picture somewhere that you feel calm, peaceful, and relaxed. This can be a place with which you are very familiar or one you can imagine easily. It should be somewhere that brings you good and comfortable feelings. Where is this place? (It could be the beach, the mountains, the woods, your front porch, etc.)

_____

_____

_____

Sight: What do you see? What about this view is pleasant to you? What do you like about what you are seeing there? (You might be looking at waves in the ocean, a beautiful mountain view, tall green trees, flowers in your yard, etc.)

_____

_____

_____

Smell: Breathe in and out slowly and deeply. What do you smell? (Maybe suntan lotion and saltwater, fresh mountain air, the aroma of fresh pine, your neighbor barbecuing, etc.)

_____

_____

_____

Touch: What are you touching? What sensations do you feel? (Perhaps gritty sand and heat from the sun, cool mountain breezes, crunchy leaves under your feet, the wicker of your porch swing, etc.)

_____

_____

_____

Taste: What do you taste? (Maybe salty seawater on your lips, clean cold water from a mountain spring, berries from the woods, sweet tea on your porch, etc.)

_____

_____

_____

Other details: What else do you notice around you? The more detail you can add to your imagery, the more effective it will be as a mindfulness tool. Try to weave in as many details as possible. Linger with this imagery for a while. Enter this scene in your mind and place yourself fully within it. Take your time. When you're done spending time in the place you chose, you can leave it the same way you entered it (e.g., through a door, on a trail).

_____

_____

_____

The more you practice this, the more effective it will be as a mindful exercise. You will find that you no longer need this worksheet as a reference and are able to bring up this imagery in rich detail whenever you need a refreshing mental (and physical) break.

MEDITATION

Most of us have heard of meditation and have a sense of what it is. The dictionary describes it as "contemplation, musing, consideration, reflection, deliberation, thinking, or introspection." Whereas meditation has similarities to these activities, it also has many unique qualities.

Meditation is a focused practice of sustained attention. Given enough practice, people can find significant benefits in peace of mind, contentment, relaxation, and reduced pain. They will catastrophize less and find relief from the rumination and pessimism that often accompany chronic pain. Their pain will be less intense due to distraction and engagement in other thoughts. Meditation also reduces reactivity and allows for calmer responses.

We can help people with chronic pain develop a meditation practice that will benefit them by reducing their pain and their responses to it. Meditation works well when people intentionally set aside time to focus attention moment by moment on some aspect of their experience and gently bring their mind back to that focus when thoughts wander (as they always do).

The following exercise will be helpful as you work with your clients in pain to move them toward a regular meditation practice.

Meditation

As you think about your life with chronic pain, you've probably wondered what you might do that will help you feel relief. Meditation is a very effective way to change how your body responds to pain. This worksheet will help you get started meditating. As you practice this, you'll find that the benefits become much more obvious and clear to you.

There are countless ways that you can approach meditation. This is one approach to try. You can always experiment with different styles of meditation until you find what fits best with your personal preferences.

- Set aside some time where you won't be interrupted.

- Minimize distractions (e.g., people, TV, music).

- Select a spot that is private and comfortable for you.

- Get comfortable. You can sit on a cushy chair, lie on the floor or a couch, or relax in a recliner.

- Close your eyes or rest your gaze on something that you like to look at.

- Breathe gently in and out, gradually slowing your breathing. Feel the breath going in and out of your nose. Notice your body relaxing.

- You may choose to direct your focus on any number of things
  - Your breathing
  - Something you're looking at (e.g., a candle, a soothing scene)
  - A word, thought, or phrase (e.g., "I'm peaceful," "I'm relaxed," "I'm content")

- Notice your breathing become slow and deep. Your thoughts will drift. When they do, gently bring your attention back to the present.

- Do this for several minutes.

- When you are ready, gently bring your awareness back to the present. Slowly return from your relaxed state of being.

Take note of improvements in how you are feeling, both mentally and physically. Once you get the hang of this, practice, practice, practice. The more frequently you do it, the more easily you will be able to bring on this feeling of calmness and peace. With more practice, you'll notice that your pain is less of a problem and that you feel more content and at ease.

PROGRESSIVE MUSCLE RELAXATION

Progressive Muscle Relaxation (PMR) is a great way to help people achieve a relaxed physical state, reducing tension in muscles. PMR is a structured way to have clients focus on different parts of the body while tensing and relaxing sets of muscles. People often aren't even aware of tightness in their bodies until they do this exercise.

PMR directly impacts some of the issues that people with chronic pain experience as a result of pain. Muscles tighten in response to pain. Protective movement patterns lead to discomfort and further pain and tightness. Chronic pain leads to muscle tension, and the reverse is also true—muscle tension leads to chronic pain. We can replace the term *chronic pain* with *emotional distress* and have another valid truth. Emotional distress leads to muscle tension, and muscle tension leads to emotional distress.

Going over the following worksheet with your clients and actually doing a PMR exercise with them will demonstrate how simple it is to do this activity on their own.

Exercise

Progressive Muscle Relaxation

Most of us aren't aware of the amount of tension we carry in our bodies. Progressive Muscle Relaxation (PMR) will give you some experience in relaxing those areas of tightness, tension, and stress. Following are some ideas you can use as you begin to practice PMR.

• Find a comfortable, quiet place and set aside a few minutes to do the exercise without interruption. Sit comfortably with your feet on the floor.

• Do some relaxation breathing until you start to feel calm and relaxed.

• Use a similar approach for each of the following muscle groups, repeating on the left and right sides of your body. Flex and tense the muscle, hold it for a few seconds, take a deep breath and release that breath, paying attention to how the muscle feels as you relax it.

- Feet

- Calves

- Thighs

- Abdomen

- Chest

- Shoulders

- Upper arms

- Lower arms

- Hands, fingers, and wrists

- Neck

- Face and jaw

- Forehead

When you've gone through all of these muscles groups (on both your right and left sides), notice the relaxation you feel in your body. Take a moment to notice your level of emotional stress and tension as well. Enjoy the feeling you now have in your body and with your emotions.

Key Points about Mindfulness for Chronic Pain

There is a robust body of evidence that supports mindful approaches to chronic pain. As you support your clients in developing these tools, remind them that developing new habits and patterns takes time and practice. The benefits they experience will likely be what keeps them engaged in mindfulness techniques.

- **Mindfulness practices** are proven to be effective in the treatment of chronic pain. They sooth reactivity to pain, enhance a sense of calm, and change the body's functioning.

- These tools boost the **parasympathetic nervous system**, allowing it to override the **sympathetic nervous system**. This will slow breathing, calm the heart rate, and minimize the physical manifestations of stress.

- **Breathing** from the diaphragm is easily learned, and with practice can become a powerful and simple intervention for those with chronic pain.

- Using **imagery** stimulates the senses and grounds people in ways that reduce chronic pain.

- **Meditation** is a habit that can be tailored to the preferences of the individual. It can be used in any setting at any time, and has robust evidence supporting its efficacy.

- **Progressive Muscle Relaxation** can be used at any time of day, with many people reporting good results when used at night for sleep problems.

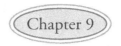
Chapter 9

Cognitive-Behavioral Interventions

> *"Pain is never permanent."*
> —Saint Teresa of Avila

Some of the most effective approaches to treat chronic pain are based in CBT. These approaches are straightforward, clear, and client-led. CBT interventions are proven to be helpful for those with chronic pain, making them an excellent treatment choice. CBT helps people look at their thoughts, identify distortions, and modify them into more productive, accurate, and helpful thoughts.

> CBT helps people look at their thoughts, identify distortions, and modify them into more productive, accurate, and helpful thoughts.

The basic premise of CBT is that situations and events don't *cause* our feelings and reactions; it's our thoughts about the situations and events that cause our distress. How we feel is strongly influenced by what we think. When we can help people think differently about their pain experience, we can dramatically reduce how much pain they feel. The following image offers a simple description of how this works.

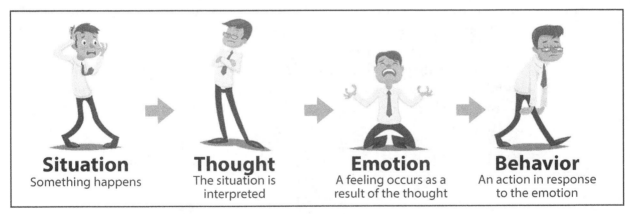

Situation
Something happens

Thought
The situation is interpreted

Emotion
A feeling occurs as a result of the thought

Behavior
An action in response to the emotion

You can see the impact that our thoughts have on our emotions and behavior. First we have a **situation**, event, or trigger. This can be anything that is stressful or upsetting. For people with chronic pain, it may be a physical sensation of pain, discomfort, or an emotional upset or stressor.

The **thought** about pain sensations determines someone's emotions and behaviors. Let's say a person with chronic pain wakes up in the middle of the night with a headache ... again. The person may have thoughts that aren't helpful. Maybe they think, "I'll never fall back asleep. I'll have a horrible day at work tomorrow because I'll be so tired. Why does this keep happening? Why can't my doctors fix what's wrong with me? I'll never get better!" And on and on and on.

It's easy to anticipate where these thoughts might lead. It's likely that the person in chronic pain is now going to feel certain **emotions** as a result of those thoughts. Some of these could include pessimism, hopelessness, sadness, frustration, and other unhelpful emotions.

These thoughts and feelings are going to lead to certain **behaviors.** Think for a moment about what behaviors you might expect given the example. It's reasonable to think that the person may start to worry, which certainly isn't sleep-inducing. The person may become less active, fearing that movement will make the pain worse. Maybe the person will call in sick for work the next day or cancel something that was planned because of the fear that the headache will worsen.

Because of central sensitization, our negative thoughts and emotions actually make the physical pain worse as well.

> The bottom line is that it's not the pain sensations themselves that determine suffering, but our interpretation of those sensations.

Consider the following example of pain and how our thoughts shape our pain experience. Imagine that someone comes up to you and punches you in the face, hard. Your nose is bloodied, maybe broken, and you may have been knocked to the floor. The pain is intense, and your mind is spinning. Your most pressing thought is probably related to how much pain you're in. The thought may be, "This pain is horrible! My nose may be broken! Look at all that blood! I can't believe how much my face hurts!"

Now picture a boxing match. A boxer gets punched in the face, hard. The boxer's nose is bloodied, maybe broken, and the boxer may have been knocked to the ground. Here's where the pain experience differs, and it's all due to the thoughts around the pain. The boxer is fired up and focused. The pain may even pump more energy into their body. In this case, the thoughts may be, "Wow! That was a strong punch! I'm going to get up and do what I'm trained to do. This is not going to set me back. I'm going to come back and win!"

The intense focus and purpose in what the boxer is doing distracts attention away from the pain and keeps their attention focused on the competition. Without that kind of focus, we can end up solely focusing on the pain. CBT interventions can be used to help people reshape their thoughts, which leads to a different emotional response and aids in the formation of new habits and behaviors.

ABC MODEL

The ABC model is a basic CBT intervention and is foundational to the other tools we discuss in this chapter. It offers a way to help people identify the thoughts that are causing them trouble

You can use the worksheet on page 102 as a strong visual aid that helps your clients see their own thought patterns. This worksheet helps people understand the importance that their thoughts play in the experience of chronic pain. It may be useful to first do this worksheet together with a client and then give them some blank worksheets to do later on their own.

Here are a few ideas about how to use this with people. You can explain very simply that it isn't the things that happen that cause us to be upset, it's how we think about those things that trips us up. Introduce this as a simple exercise to illustrate how we do that. You can give people the sheet of paper and a pen and have them fill it out themselves, which may add to their sense of "owning" what they come up with.

Ask your client to describe an upsetting event, preferably somewhat recent. Use that in the first column. At this point, you are just trying to demonstrate the exercise, so any example will do. The example might be a recent pain episode, a fight with a family member, an issue with a boss, or anything that is relevant for the person.

Once the trigger event is filled in, move to the second column. Have the client clearly spell out what they were thinking and telling themselves about the event. These thoughts can be wide ranging, and they are all worth writing down. You may need to remind the person to focus on their thoughts, not their feelings. Thoughts could be "Nobody can fix me," "I think this will never end," "I know I'll never get better," or "Nobody listens to me." Once the person is done with that column, it's time to look at the impact of those thoughts.

The third column is where the person lists feelings and reactions experienced as a result of their thoughts. These could include sadness, anger, frustration, loneliness, kicking a wall, crying, or any other emotion or reaction.

The pattern is now down on paper and describes the person's reality. Next, you want to take another stab at the experience from a different perspective. Using the same trigger event, have the person cross out the middle column, which includes the thoughts they had about the event. Have them come up with a new, more helpful set of thoughts they could have. They could say, "Maybe I'll feel better tomorrow," "It's possible the person didn't mean to do what they did to me," "Maybe I can figure out how to handle this," and so on. If your client gets stuck, you might gently nudge them with a couple of prompts, but this really needs to be their material.

After the client has crossed out the feelings and reactions they originally wrote down, have them look at the new list of thoughts they could choose to have. If they choose to have those thoughts instead of the original ones, what feelings would they have? They can now develop a revised list of feelings and reactions they could have as a result of having new and different thoughts. The goal of this activity is to assist people in understanding that when they choose to have different thoughts, they will end up having different feelings.

Worshseet

ABC Model

You can use this worksheet to help identify your thoughts and how they impact your feelings and reactions. Start with an event, trigger, or stressor. Write that down in the first column. The second column is where you'll jot down your thoughts and what you were telling yourself about that event. Next, fill in the third column with how you felt and reacted—what you did.

The next part of the exercise is to play with what might happen if you decided to think some different thoughts about the trigger. Cross out the thoughts that you listed the first time through. Under them, write out a different set of thoughts and things you could tell yourself. Focus on thoughts that are true, accurate, and new.

Once you've developed a new set of thoughts, move on to the third column and cross out the feelings that you already wrote down there. Look at the new set of thoughts you developed and ponder how you might feel if you thought them to yourself. Those feelings are sure to be different than the first set of feelings. You'll probably see that when you *think* about a trigger differently, you will end up *feeling* differently about it.

Activating Event, Trigger, Stressor	Beliefs/Thoughts	Consequences, Feelings, Behaviors
What happened?	*What did you tell yourself?* *What were you thinking?*	*How did you feel?* *What did you do?*

Case Example

Mark – The Reluctant Client

Mark came in for services at the age of 43. He had been in pain for the past seven years, ever since he had a car accident that led to back pain. Since that time, he had only worked intermittently, feeling he could no longer do the construction work that he used to. After he developed chronic pain, he could only do odd jobs for neighbors and friends when he was feeling up to it. He was resentful and less active and reported that all of this had contributed to his experiencing depression.

"I feel horrible, my back hurts all the time, and I know I'll never be back to normal. Whenever I try to do something I hurt even worse. My partner is frustrated and doesn't understand that when I hurt, I just don't feel like doing anything," he lamented. Clearly, he had some fixed thoughts that were impacting his ability to get better. *"I've been to doctors and counselors in the past, and it did me no good,"* he continued.

At first, Mark was reluctant to engage in therapy. He was offended that his doctor had suggested it but decided to give it one last shot. After a thorough assessment and consultation with his physician, we got to work.

Several CBT exercises seemed to help shift his firmly held beliefs, and he was able to look at his thought distortions more clearly. Our first intervention was to complete the "ABC" worksheet (which looks at "A"—an activating event, "B"—beliefs, and "C"—consequences of those beliefs). Following is what Mark's worksheet looked like once we had worked through it:

Activating Event, Trigger, Stressor	Beliefs/Thoughts	Consequences, Feelings, Behaviors
What happened?	*What did you tell yourself?* *What were you thinking?*	*How did you feel?* *What did you do?*
I woke up in the middle of the night and my back was hurting	• This is terrible • I'll be so tired tomorrow • My doctors will never figure this out • I'll never get better • This could be cancer	• Couldn't sleep • Worried • Mad at doctors • Scared
Now with revised thoughts . . .	• I've had worse back pain • Maybe I can take some Tylenol • I could try that relaxation technique that I learned • Maybe I can sleep in a little bit	*Now check out the new feelings and reactions:* • I stayed in bed—at least my body was resting • I was calmer and less upset • I wasn't as scared • After a little bit I was able to fall asleep

Once Mark had gotten the hang of how to complete this exercise, he was able to do it on his own. He came in to a later session and shared what he had come up with while using this worksheet for a different issue. He reported that his activating event was when his partner would "yell and holler" at him when he couldn't participate in whatever it was she wanted him to do. When asked what he felt or did when that happened (consequences), he explained that he felt "angry, frustrated, helpless, sad, and lonely" and would "yell back" or withdraw and leave the room. As we looked at the middle column (beliefs), it took him several moments to ponder his answer: *"I probably tell myself that she doesn't care enough to understand, she'll never get it and that she thinks I'm a loser and that I don't have anything to contribute anymore."*

As we moved into considering what he could tell himself that's different from that, it took him a few minutes to figure out some alternative thoughts: *"Maybe I could tell myself that she's scared, she's worn out, I do contribute by watching our kids while she works, and that maybe she's missing what she used to have."*

At this point, his mood had visibly softened. As he considered how he might feel and what he might do if he chose to tell himself these revised thoughts, he admitted that he could feel less angry, more understanding of her, and less reactive. *"I probably wouldn't yell back or take it as personally,"* he decided. *"And I might feel less alone with my frustration."*

THOUGHT DISTORTIONS

Identifying distorted thoughts and cognitions is at the heart of CBT and is relevant to our treatment of people with chronic pain. Clients often tell themselves things that aren't actually true or are distorted, and these skewed beliefs negatively impact their ability to get better. These distortions often hold steady over time and become long-term beliefs that people can hold onto with a firm grip.

Once we help our clients identify their thought distortions, we can help them assess how accurate, true, and helpful those thoughts are (or aren't). The following worksheet can be used to help people see what their most common thought distortions are.

One way to introduce this exercise is to issue a caution about the perils of believing everything you think. Just because something seems true doesn't make it so. Most of us believe a lot of things that aren't accurate, and it is helpful to pay careful attention to our beliefs so we can modify them as needed.

Thought Distortions

We often have distortions in how we think about things. Since these thinking patterns involve mistakes in how we perceive situations, they lead to automatic negative thoughts that then increase our emotional upset and physical pain. Look over this list and see which of these thinking errors you make most often. Add in your own examples.

1. All-or-Nothing Thinking

You see things in black-or-white, either-or categories instead of in terms of degree. If a situation falls short of perfection, it's a failure.

Example: "I can only be happy if I am pain-free."

My example _____

_____

2. Overgeneralizing

You may see a certain situation as a never-ending pattern—one that happens over and over again. You view one or two bad events as an endless pattern of defeat.

Example: "I tried doing exercises for my back pain before and it didn't help then, so it isn't going to help now."

My example _____

_____

3. Mental Filtering

You focus only on the negative aspects of a situation and ignore positive aspects.

Example: "I tried walking but couldn't go very far at all before I started hurting."

My example _____

_____

4. Discounting the Positive

Positive experiences or achievements are discounted or dismissed or don't count. This entails focusing on the bad and disqualifying the good.

Example: "So what if I'm doing more—I'm still in pain."

My example _____

_____

5. Jumping to Conclusions

You may make assumptions or interpret situations negatively without any facts to support the assumptions, or you might make negative conclusions about events that aren't based on facts.

Example: "I feel useless, so I have no value."

My example _____

_____

6. Mind Reading

Without checking it out, you may assume that you know what someone is thinking and why they are thinking it.

Example: "I know people think I'm faking my pain."

My example _____

_____

7. Fortune Telling

You predict that things will turn out badly without any evidence.

Example: "I could try that new therapy my doctor told me about, but I know it won't help."

My example _____

_____

8. Catastrophizing

You tend to expect the worst possible outcome, while at the same time minimizing your ability to cope. This is a belief that the worst possible thing will happen.

Example: "When my pain is so bad, I know I'll never get any better."

My example _____

_____

9. Emotional Reasoning

There is a tendency to assume that negative feelings reflect the way things actually are.

Example: "I feel useless, so I AM useless."

My example _____

_____

10. Labeling

This is a form of all-or-nothing thinking in which you deal with mistakes by attaching general labels to yourself or others.

Example: "I'm a failure and a loser because I can't do any activity at all."

My example _____

_____

11. Personalization

You assume full responsibility for situations and problems that are not completely under your control.

Example: "I know that I caused my problem to get worse because I started that new job that I hate."

My example _____

_____

12. Control Error

You believe that other people cause you to feel certain ways.

Example: "My mom makes me so angry that she is making my pain worse."

My example _____

_____

13. Should/Shouldn't Statements

You tell yourself how you ought to act, think, or feel or how other people or things should be. Often this is expressed as what "must" happen.

Example: "My doctor should be able to cure my pain."

My example _____

_____

Case Example

Mark – Continued

Let's check in on Mark again. As we worked on thought distortions, it didn't take him long at all to pick the one he used most. He identified overgeneralizing as his go-to distortion. As if to demonstrate the accuracy of his choice, he added, *"I do that all the time!"* His example had to do with his partner again. He explained it like this: *"I try to describe to her what this pain has done to me, and she never gets it. It seems like she's always mad and she never feels any other emotions—especially compassion or understanding."*

It's unlikely that those were the *only* emotions his partner *ever* felt. It was worthwhile for Mark to take the time to carefully assess the truth and helpfulness of his fixed thoughts. He ended up being able to modify those thoughts and shift them to thoughts that were more true and beneficial to him.

AUTOMATIC NEGATIVE THOUGHTS—ANTS!

Most of us have automatic negative thoughts (ANTS). We gain control and are able to make positive changes when we can recognize what our ANTS are and decide how we want to change them. The process is fairly simple, though not always easy to carry out. The solution may be clear, but changing entrenched thought patterns can be difficult.

Automatic negative thoughts are usually spontaneous, repetitive, and believable to us. We see them as plausible and reasonable. They are specific, habitual, and involuntary. This can be a form of negative self-talk that we aren't even aware of, and these thought patterns can have a strong negative pull on us. These thoughts need to be brought into the light where we can see how to best modify them.

Automatic negative thoughts often reflect critical beliefs about the self, such as, "I'm so stupid," "I'll never be able to manage my pain," or "I'm worthless because I can't do more for my family." ANTS can actually become entrenched and somewhat fixed. It usually takes targeted interventions to reshape those thoughts in ways that are more helpful and accurate.

One intervention that's valuable for people with chronic pain is to use the following worksheet to help identify their ANTS, do a brief review of the evidence for and against the thoughts, look for alternative viewpoints, and come up with revised thoughts.

Automatic Negative Thoughts—ANTS!

Automatic negative thought

_____

_____

Testing the automatic thought

What is the evidence that supports this belief?

_____

_____

What is the evidence against this belief?

_____

_____

What are the errors in my thinking (cognitive distortions)?

_____

_____

What is an alternative viewpoint?

_____

_____

What can I do to help myself?

_____

_____

What is the effect of my thinking?

_____

_____

Revised thought

_____

_____

Case Example

Mark – Continued

Now let's consider how this might look for Mark. This may help give you an idea of the types of things that may come up through this exercise.

Mark's automatic negative thought: *I'm never going to get better. I've had pain for years and I'll always be miserable.*

Testing the automatic thought

What is the evidence that supports this belief? *I hurt almost all the time. I'm never completely pain free; I'm never at a zero on the pain scale. I've had chronic pain for seven years now, and nobody has been able to help me.*

What's the evidence against this belief? *Well, I guess there are times when the pain level is lower. Sometimes I can get out and do things, but I still hurt. I can't do the things I used to do, but sometimes I feel a little bit better. There might be a few options for treatment that I haven't tried yet.*

What are the errors in my thinking (cognitive distortions)? *If I review that worksheet we did on thought distortions, it looks like I might be doing overgeneralizing—again.*

What is an alternative viewpoint? *I could try to make some small changes that don't make my pain worse, and I could start noticing times that I don't hurt as badly.*

What can I do to help myself? *I might try to follow my program more closely. I could do more to increase my activity level (slowly), and I could try to see my friends more.*

What is the effect of my thinking? *It keeps me on the couch. I think it also makes me more sad and lonely. It also makes me irritable with my partner.*

Revised thought: *It's possible that I could see some improvement. Even if I have pain, I don't have to be miserable and hopeless. Maybe if I do more I'll feel better.*

DOWNWARD ARROW

This is a process that helps people tease out a core belief that is causing distress or discomfort. People often feel unsettled and bothered by things, and they can't figure out why they are having such a big impact on them. They're often looking at these things superficially and really need to get at their core beliefs. The following worksheet can help with this process.

This can be a powerful tool in helping people look more deeply at their core beliefs and how they boost or inhibit progress toward greater health and well-being. This is something you might want to try when you have gained a client's trust and they feel somewhat comfortable disclosing thoughts that can be fairly intimate and personal. This can stir up a lot of emotion and expose thoughts that people weren't even aware they had.

Downward Arrow

Downward arrow will help you figure out what's at the core of some of your upsetting responses to things. You may be looking at things as they appear to be on the surface, and you may benefit from looking more deeply at what is stirring up your reactions.

What is a thought that's been bothering you?

_____

_____

What does this mean about you?

_____

_____

What does this mean about you?

_____

_____

What does this mean about you?

_____

_____

(Repeat until you feel you've reached your core belief)

My core belief:

_____

_____

Case Example

Mark – Continued

Let's walk through the previous "Downward Arrow" worksheet and see how it looked when Mark was finished with it.

What's a thought that's been bothering you? *I feel like I caused my pain to be worse by not taking better care of myself.*

What does this mean about you? *That I don't have any self-control.*

What does this mean about you? *This means I'm weak and not committed.*

What does this mean about you? *That I must not care enough about myself to try.*

My core belief: *I am not worth anything.*

CATASTROPHIZING

We can think of catastrophizing as jumping to the worst possible outcome without cause. This can look like an illogical leap that only causes disruption. Pain catastrophizing is almost universal for people with chronic pain. Unfortunately, it leads to horrible outcomes if it is not interrupted.

> Pain catastrophizing is almost universal for people with chronic pain. Unfortunately, it leads to horrible outcomes if it is not interrupted.

Pain catastrophizing is linked to greater pain intensity, worse outcomes after surgery, longer hospital stays, more depression, and a *reduced* response to opioids. People who catastrophize are more likely to develop chronic pain after injury or surgery. It's widely known that pain catastrophizing is a more impactful factor in pain outcomes than disease or pain condition.

Pain catastrophizing often includes three key features: rumination, helplessness, and magnification. People ruminate about their pain—it consumes a great deal of thought, time, and energy. This is often accompanied by a sense of helplessness. Magnification is tied to this, as pain looms large and dominates so many facets of life.

We often see that people who catastrophize tend to overestimate risk and danger while underestimating their resources and ability to cope. We want to help people form a more realistic appraisal of risk, danger, and their own coping abilities and resources.

The worksheet on page 114 can be useful in helping people confront their fears and tap into their strengths and resources.

Completing this worksheet helps in several ways. There is a benefit to having people talk about (and write down) their worst fear. Confronting fears, even when they are not the worst ones, and writing them down and talking with you about them is significant.

This process helps diminish the potency of the fears. We are also helping people form a more realistic appraisal of the likely outcome, identify coping skills, and weaken the grip that this fear has on them.

Having people rate the likelihood of this feared event happening (second column) puts a numeric value down on paper. When clients are able to identify an outcome that is more likely to happen (last column) than their feared outcome (second column), this clearly demonstrates a major benefit of the exercise.

When we ask clients what they would do and how they would cope if this feared event happened (third column), we are helping them identify their own resources and external supports. When they take time to identify their internal and external resources, they are empowered to view a scary event with less fear and a more realistic and accurate assessment of risk.

Cognitive-behavioral approaches have been shown to be powerful and effective tools to help people with chronic pain change their thinking patterns, identify thought distortions, modify automatic negative thoughts, get at their core beliefs, decatastrophize, and gain more realistic ideas about and control over their pain.

Worksheet

Decatastrophizing

My worst fear	How likely is this? (0–100)	What would I do if it did happen? How would I cope?	What is the most likely outcome?

Case Example
Mark – Continued

Here's an example of how the "Decatastrophizing" worksheet might look when completed by our friend Mark.

My worst fear: *My pain has been so bad that now I think I must have cancer.*

How likely is this? (0–100): *It seems like cancer is the only thing that could cause this much pain for so long. I think it could be 80–90.*

What would I do if it did happen? How would I cope? *I hate to even think about this because I'm afraid it will make it come true. But if I did have cancer, I guess I'd get a thorough medical evaluation, testing, and treatment recommendations. If I had to, I would probably do chemo, surgery, or radiation. I'd get counseling. I could join a support group, either in person or online. If I had to have surgery, I guess I'd do that. I could talk with my best friend—she went through cancer a while back.*

What's the most likely outcome? *I probably don't have cancer after all.*

Key Points of Cognitive-Behavioral Interventions

- **Cognitive-behavioral approaches** are proven to be the most helpful ways to reduce chronic pain and the associated suffering. We know that it isn't just chronic pain that makes people feel bad; it's their thoughts about the pain that increase both pain and emotional distress.

- The **ABC exercise** is a clear way to help people identify their thoughts that contribute to their physical pain and upsetting emotional reactions.

- Helping people identify their **thought distortions** enables them to shift their problematic patterns of thinking. As they notice these thinking habits they will be able to modify those patterns and reduce their impact.

- **Automatic negative thoughts (ANTS!)** are spontaneous, believable, repetitive thoughts. They are often critical and pessimistic, preventing people from thriving. Adjusting those negative thought patterns can dramatically change people's responses to pain.

- **Downward arrow** is an exercise that helps people expose themselves to a feared thought and gets to a core belief that the person may not even be consciously aware of.

- **Decatastrophizing** is one of the most important tools we can offer people in pain. Catastrophizing is almost universal with chronic pain, and by giving people the ability to stop catastrophizing we arm them with an essential tool for recovery.

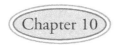

Essential Treatment Components

> *"Vodka does not ease back pain.*
> *But it does get your mind off it."*
> —*Fuzzy Zoeller*

We've spent some time on mindfulness and cognitive-behavioral approaches to treating pain, and there are many other approaches to choose from as you treat people with pain. In this chapter you'll find a variety of additional options to strengthen your treatment results.

PAIN TRACKING

People with chronic pain will find tremendous benefit in tracking their pain and their emotions related to it. Examining pain and feelings helps people see the relationship between physical and emotional components of pain.

People can note as much detail as they want as they log their pain. Not only can they note the intensity on a 0 to 10 scale, they can further describe the details of the pain sensations. Sensations may include pounding, aching, dull, throbbing, sharp, pulsing, burning, and tightness.

Emotions linked to the pain may include sadness, anger, frustration, and anxiety. The feelings can lead to increased pain, and they may also be a result of pain.

Your clients may also want to track thoughts about their pain. "I'll never get better!" "This is just horrible," "I'm so frustrated with how little I can do now!" are all common thoughts of people with chronic pain.

The following worksheet helps give structure to the process of tracking the pain experience.

Pain Tracking

Tracking your pain and its related emotions and thoughts can be a practical way to note progress and growth. Consider using this worksheet as you get started in treatment.

Date	Time	Pain (0–10)	Emotions/Feelings	Thoughts	What I Did that Helped

As you track your physical pain, emotions, and thoughts, you may start to see patterns emerge. This will give you some important guidance as you learn to observe and respond to your pain differently.

PLEASANT ACTIVITY SCHEDULING

Sadly, one of the things that falls by the wayside for most people with chronic pain is doing pleasant, enjoyable activities. People are often less socially involved and less physically active. This may be due to physical discomfort and limitations and mood changes related to living with pain. When people are depressed, anxious, and discouraged, they are much less likely to take part in things they used to enjoy.

People with pain often need some prompting to re-engage with activities they used to enjoy and take pleasure in. This can shift pessimism to optimism and inactivity to movement. We can help people come up with doable ideas for activities in which they are likely to take part. Use the following worksheet to guide your clients as they begin this process.

Pleasant Activity Scheduling

You may find that over time you've been less involved in activities you used to enjoy. This may be due to physical pain or emotional challenges. You can gradually reintroduce those pleasant activities into your life by taking the following steps:

1. Brainstorm a list of activities, hobbies, and activities you used to enjoy or that you still take part in. Even if you can't do the activity in quite the same way because of your pain, write it down anyway. Make the list as long as it needs to be and don't rule anything out at this point. What are some of those activities?

   _____

   _____

   _____

2. Which of those activities sound appealing to you? Which ones are you most likely to do now?

   _____

   _____

   _____

3. There may be some things on your list that you aren't able to do in the same way you used to. What adjustments could you make in those activities that would enable you to take part in them now, even in a modified way?

   _____

   _____

   _____

4. Try getting specific and detailed in how you might take part in some of these activities. When might you do them? With whom? Where?

   _____

   _____

   _____

As you start to do some of these activities, keep track of what is working for you and what you enjoy. Consider this a work in progress and make changes whenever you need to.

TIME-BASED PACING

Accomplishing tasks in a way that doesn't contribute to a physical setback can be a challenge for people with chronic pain. Sometimes they overdo it on a day when they're having less pain and then they have a hard time recovering from doing too much. Some think they need to push through their pain and end up feeling much worse for it. After a lengthy recovery time, they may do the same thing again because now they feel that they are behind and need to catch up.

There are some effective ways to work around this. One of the best ways to approach task completion is to shift the focus from working on a job until it's done to working for predetermined segments of time with rest periods in between. Thus, time-based pacing is a simple concept. Instead of looking at a task and deciding to take a break when the job is halfway done, the person can decide to take a break every half hour. This pacing helps prevent a pain flare and the need for a lengthy recovery that comes from being too ambitious and unrealistic.

The cycle of work and rest is much more even and predictable with time-based pacing than it is when people work through the pain and push themselves in spite of discomfort. Building in rest at certain intervals ends up being a much more productive approach.

The following worksheet can help your clients use time-based pacing effectively.

Time-Based Pacing

You may have noticed that when you have a task to do, you push on to finish it even if you are going to have a flare-up of your pain. You may believe that it has to get done and if you're feeling better that day you should just keep working until it's finished. That's an approach that can actually make things worse, causing a prolonged recovery time as you get over the pain that is now worse from doing the job.

This worksheet can help you use a different approach called time-based pacing. If you take breaks at scheduled times, you'll end up needing less time to recover from the job.

Think about a task that's in front of you and how this new approach might work.

• Think of a task that you need to complete that could increase your pain.

_____

_____

_____

• Consider how long you can work on this task without it increasing your pain. That is the amount of time you can aim to work before taking a break. Make it short enough that you don't think it will cause any increase in your pain. How long is that time period?

_____

_____

_____

• If you take a break at that period of time, how long will you need to rest before you start up again?

_____

_____

_____

Try this approach with this task and with any other projects that you have coming up. Adjust your time estimates as needed. See if you can engage in a regular rhythm of work and rest without increasing your pain.

SLEEP CHALLENGES

Sleep problems are almost universal in people with chronic pain. Pain impacts sleep, and sleep deprivation worsens pain. It's imperative that we work with our clients to help improve their quality of sleep. The use of sleep medications is generally discouraged because of their addictive properties. A behavioral treatment called CBT-I (cognitive-behavioral therapy for insomnia) has proven to be effective in helping people normalize their sleep patterns and get the restful and restorative sleep they so desperately need.

The Insomnia Severity Index is a tool that can help gauge the impact of a client's sleep issues. It is quick to administer and easy to score. It gives a snapshot of the client's sleep challenges and helps guide us as we intervene to establish healthy sleep routines.

There are several things that impact sleep for those with chronic pain. Pain is taxing on the body and, ironically, that fatigue works against falling asleep easily at night. Some people find that as the activity and distraction

> Pain is taxing on the body and, ironically, that fatigue works against falling asleep easily at night.

of the day winds down and they're in bed alone with their thoughts, they tend to focus on their sensations of pain. Anxiety may build and they may notice physical discomfort more. Chronic sleeplessness actually increases pain sensitivity in the body. Pain may also make it more difficult to fall asleep when people wake up in the middle of the night.

As you may know from times when you yourself had sleep issues (e.g., with a new baby, cramming for exams), there are lots of consequences of poor sleep. People with sleeplessness may experience concentration challenges, irritability, muscle aches and headaches, low energy, and fatigue.

There are a couple of factors to assess when talking about sleep problems with clients who have chronic pain. You want to consider the possibility of obstructive sleep apnea (OSA) and refer them to a specialist as needed. The risk of OSA increases with the use of opioids and muscle relaxers. If a person with chronic pain has become less active and more sedentary, they may develop obesity, thus raising their risk of OSA.

Healthy sleep allows for physical restoration, which is imperative in improving chronic pain. It also reduces pain sensitivity and helps tissue heal. When talking with someone who has trouble sleeping, there are several areas on which to focus.

- Alcohol use before bed: Alcohol use may contribute to sleep problems. People who drink before bed may fall asleep more quickly, but the alcohol can lead to lighter sleep and middle-of-the-night awakenings.
- Caffeine use: Caffeine stays in the body for nine to ten hours after ingestion, so it can have an impact on sleep. Even caffeine ingested in the afternoon may impair a person's ability to fall asleep easily at night.
- Daytime activity: Increasing daytime activity can help increase tiredness and physical fatigue, both of which help people fall asleep better at night.

- Daytime bed use: It is helpful to limit daytime bed use and lying down during the day. Lying down increases the possibility of napping, which makes it harder to fall asleep at night. Daytime bed use also can contribute to the bed being associated with being awake rather than being asleep, and it can allow the person to be less active.

- Eating and drinking: It's generally a good idea to avoid heavy eating just before bed. Digestion slows at night, making for fuller sensations. Acid reflux may occur and cause discomfort. It's also suggested that people limit their fluid intake to reduce the need to get up at night to urinate.

- Medication: Medications can contribute to sleep problems, so it's important to work with the person's primary care physician to look at the impact of medication regimens. Opioid medications may cause drowsiness, but they end up interfering with quality sleep.

- Routine: Most people see improvement in their sleep when they maintain a consistent bedtime and wakeup time. Varying those times by very much can disrupt the person's ability to develop good patterns of sleep.

- Stimulus control: This is an important part of the CBT-I protocol to help people shift their sleep patterns. Suggestions include only using the bed for sleeping or sex, only going to bed when sleepy (as opposed to when just "worn out" or when "it's time" to go to bed), getting up if you're awake for 20 minutes rather than continuing to lie in bed, avoiding naps, and establishing a regular sleep-wake cycle.

INCREASING ACTIVITY LEVEL

Increasing activity and movement is one of the core interventions to use with a client who has chronic pain. Most everyone with chronic pain is less physically active, which leads to deconditioning. When you can get someone moving more, you are helping them make positive changes to both their body and mind.

There are several things you can do to get your clients moving more. The goal is to get them to be active enough to see that movement isn't damaging and doesn't cause further pain. They should keep at the activity until their anxiety around it is diminished. One way to do this is to have them choose pleasurable activities that they enjoy doing and to engage in them three to four times a week. Some clients do well trying endurance activities that emphasize flexibility and strength. Tracking these activities is a proven approach, so having clients document their successes can be a great help in their progress.

FAMILY INVOLVEMENT

Chronic pain has a powerful impact on families. There are many ways that families experience the chronic pain of a relative. Family activities may be different (if they're happening at all). The person with pain may not be functioning in the same roles in the same way they used to. Sexual relationships may be damaged by the physical challenges of pain. The social life of a couple or family may take a hit as the person with pain becomes more withdrawn and less able to engage with relatives or friends. There may be a financial impact on the family if the person is not able to work in the same way or at the same income as before. Family roles may shift.

Sometimes family members just don't know how to help. They may be angry and feel guilty about being mad at someone in pain. They could resent the additional load on themselves. On the other hand, they may be overly helpful and protective of the person with pain. This may or may not be received well. Partners may be seen as punitive or as overly solicitous.

Family members may benefit from seeking help and support for themselves. It's hard to navigate all the changes that come when chronic pain intrudes on a family. Family members should keep the person with pain in charge of their own care to avoid becoming overly responsible for their progress. There's a fine line between being supportive and enabling the person with pain, preventing them from doing things for themselves. Families can encourage the person to be more actively involved in their care while working to manage their own emotional reactions (e.g., fear, anger, worry).

WORKING WITH CLIENTS ON OPIOIDS

If you treat clients with chronic pain, you will undoubtedly work with many who have been, or still are, taking opioids for their pain. As noted previously, opioids have never been shown to be beneficial when used for more than three months for chronic pain. Epidemiologic studies have shown that people on chronic opioid therapy have a poorer quality of life. It is a reasonable goal to help your clients with chronic pain understand this and motivate them to try to decrease or stop their opioid use. This should be done collaboratively with their prescriber. You will find that most prescribers know less about pain than you have already learned in this book. Prescribers get almost no education on the treatment of pain, particularly chronic pain.

> You will find that most prescribers know less about pain than you have already learned in this book.

Reducing opioid use can be a very sensitive and challenging aspect of working with people with chronic pain. Most prescribers will be excited and relieved to have you as a part of the pain treatment team. The overwhelming majority of prescribers don't like keeping people on chronic opioid therapy. However, a small subset of physicians are earning large salaries by prescribing opioids for chronic pain.

Physicians and other providers who are prescribing opioids for chronic pain should be regularly following three things with their patients: They should be regularly checking the level of pain as reported by the person; they should also be assessing their functional status and their quality of life. Current recommendations are that opioids should only be continued if all three of these areas are improving significantly. Most physicians do not measure these aspects of their patients' lives. This is something therapists can easily do in their offices. The Pain, Enjoyment of Life, and General Activity (PEG) screening tool can be helpful in this. These three major areas of life are measured for people with chronic pain. Following is the PEG assessment.

Worksheet
PEG Assessment
(Pain, Enjoyment of Life, and General Activity Level)

1. What number best describes your <u>pain on average</u> in the past week:

0	1	2	3	4	5	6	7	8	9	10

No Pain   Pain as bad as you can imagine

2. What number best describes how, during the past week, pain has interfered with your <u>enjoyment of life</u>?

0	1	2	3	4	5	6	7	8	9	10

Does not interfere   Completely interferes

3. What number best describes how, during the past week, pain has interfered with your <u>general activity</u>?

0	1	2	3	4	5	6	7	8	9	10

Does not interfere   Completely interferes

This scale can be extremely helpful to you and the prescriber to see how your client is doing on an ongoing basis. The CDC recommends continuing opioid treatment only if there is 30% improvement over baseline after starting on the medication. Often, there is an initial 30% improvement that lasts the first few weeks (the "Dorothy reaction"), then things get worse. You may not start treating the client until after they have already been on opioids, but the PEG scale is still a good general measure of how they are doing overall and how they are responding to your interventions.

It's important to remember that about 50% of people with chronic pain who do start on opioids will stop them because of side effects or lack of benefit. Of those who continue on opioids, most will report only slight improvement (about 1 point on a 0–10 scale)

> Of those who continue on opioids, most will report only slight improvement (about 1 point on a 0–10 scale) compared with placebo.

compared with placebo (Shaheed et al., 2016). Pain experts believe that it takes an improvement of about 1.5 point for the individual to notice any significant difference (Ostelo et al., 2008).

Once someone has been on opioids for more than about three months, they will not want to come off. Even though their quality of life is worse, they won't believe that they can discontinue the medication. Most have tried to reduce their dose and experienced the symptoms of opioid withdrawal, which include:

- Increased pain
- Severe anxiety and fear
- Severe depression
- Sleep disturbance

- Nausea
- Restlessness
- Inability to concentrate or think clearly

For many people, the withdrawal symptom that is the most problematic is fear. It is extremely distressing. People who have tried to reduce their dose and have experienced this fear are very reluctant to try again.

Although it is difficult, people *can* wean off opioids. Research has shown that when people with chronic pain wean off, their pain improves by about 20%. There is no set protocol for weaning. It is difficult but *not* dangerous. For people on medium to high doses of opioids, reducing the dose by 10% of the original dose each month for 10 months is reasonable. These individuals will need a lot of support during the process. Make sure the client and their family know that the process will be difficult but that once they are off these medications, they usually experience some pain relief and better quality of life.

When you work with clients who don't want to get off their opioid medications and whose doctor wants to continue prescribing, there are other measures you should consider:

- Opioids at home should be locked up. Anyone with an opioid in their home is at increased risk of home invasion and robbery. Even family members may take this medication.

- Any medications that are not used should be disposed of. Contact local law enforcement to see if there is a local mechanism to do this. The FDA and EPA both say that these medications may be flushed if unused.
- People on opioids may be impaired and should not drive. Opioids may cause significant confusion in the elderly.
- People on opioids are at a four times greater risk of falling and breaking bones. Make sure family members work to reduce fall risk.
- Monitor for new-onset depression. People on opioids are twice as likely to be depressed as people with chronic pain who aren't on opioids.
- Regularly measure their PEG scores and share these with the prescriber if they are not done there.

Opioids for chronic pain have never been shown to be effective when used for more than three months. They do increase risks and often result in worse outcomes. Your role as the therapists is to understand these effects and communicate them with people. If they decide to come off of opioids, they will ultimately feel better but will need a lot of behavioral treatment and encouragement during this frightening and difficult process.

Key Points of Essential Treatment Components

In addition to mindfulness and cognitive-behavioral approaches, we also want to look at several other **essential treatment components**. These areas are important to consider as part of a treatment plan.

- **Pain tracking** helps people become more objective about their pain and provides a written record of progress. Tracking options are generally simple and easy for clients to comply with.

- **Pleasant activity scheduling** is an important way to introduce (or re-introduce) hobbies and interests. Many people with pain have very few things in their lives that bring them joy and contentment, this exercise will help bring people in touch with those parts of their lives again.

- Using **time-based pacing** enables people to accomplish tasks without the long recovery time associated with overdoing it. This gives a structure to task accomplishment and builds success and appropriate expectations around project completion.

- One of the most important aspects of treatment is **increasing activity level**. Many people with pain avoid activity, becoming deconditioned and sedentary.

- Looking at **family dynamics** helps us factor in the various roles that family members can play while having a family member in pain. Relationships can be supported in ways that are beneficial for everyone in the family.

- For **clients on opioids** we want to be sure we are working collaboratively with the person's medical team. We can provide essential assessment of such things as pain level, quality of life, and functional status.

Chapter 11

Ethics and Pain Treatment

> *"Black patients were treated much later in their disease process. They were often not given the same kind of pain management that white patients would have gotten, and they died more often of diseases."*
> —*Rebecca Skloot*

The ethics of pain treatment are complex but are based on the four principles of medical ethics, which are:

1. Beneficence: In all that we do, we should attempt to help people.
2. Non-maleficence: In all that we do, we should try not to hurt people.
3. Autonomy: People should be able to choose their care and treatment when they are able to make these decisions.
4. Justice: Everyone is treated equally.

These principles of ethics should underlie all that we do. This chapter discusses numerous ethical issues concerning the treatment of pain. We begin by looking at medical ethics as they are applied to the overall problem of pain. We'll follow that by examining medical ethics as they apply to the treatment of pain with opioids. Following that, we discuss medical ethics and behavioral treatment of pain, concentrating on the special issues of pain in children, minorities, and the elderly.

MEDICAL ETHICS AND PAIN TREATMENT

In the United States, it is widely accepted that pain is a significant problem and that it should be addressed in a way that is beneficial and not harmful to the individual or to society. The autonomy principle of medical ethics can be problematic in pain treatment. Studies have shown that people with chronic pain develop transformations in areas of their brains that result in changes in how they perceive and react to pain. These changes also can affect their decision-making. Because of this, the issue of autonomy becomes complex. In some cases, complete autonomy is not appropriate. This particularly impacts the use of medications for pain treatment.

The ethical principle of justice becomes challenging particularly (and ironically) in the United States. The irony is that one of the richest countries in the world doesn't provide ethical pain treatment to the poor. Our market-based system of healthcare has resulted in a situation where treatment of pain and other medical conditions is preferentially provided to those with insurance or money. This is particularly significant because studies have concluded that people living in poverty have more pain than those who are more affluent. More pain with less availability of treatment results in an ethical crisis for pain treatment in the United States.

MEDICAL ETHICS AND OPIOID TREATMENT

The use of opioids for the treatment of pain is particularly problematic when we consider the ethics of pain treatment. The evidence for beneficence with opioid use for pain is weak. As noted previously, the scientific data show that that opioids are the least effective of all the oral treatments for acute pain and do not produce clinically significant reductions in chronic pain.

The evidence for maleficence with opioid treatment is much greater. In addition, there is a large *societal* maleficent impact that results in the deaths of tens of thousands of people in the United States each year.

MEDICAL ETHICS AND BEHAVIORAL TREATMENT

Based on the principles of medical ethics, counseling is likely the *most* ethical of all options for the treatment of chronic pain. In almost all cases, counseling will be beneficial and is unlikely to cause harm. The very nature of counseling and behavioral therapy involves clients having autonomy and involvement in their own care. There are still issues with justice, as those with lower socioeconomic status are less likely to receive care; however, the mental health system may do better at providing care to low-income individuals than does the rest of the medical community.

In treating chronic pain, there are additional ethical considerations we should consider. Without careful monitoring of our treatment, we can end up compromising ethical dilemmas and may do more harm than good. Let's take a look at some ethical concerns with children, the elderly, and minorities.

ETHICAL ISSUES WITH CHILDREN

Increasing numbers of children are experiencing chronic pain. There are a multitude of challenges when treating these children (and their families).

Historically, we've been challenged by recurrent pain in children. We haven't known how to measure or treat it. Very young children don't have the verbal skills to describe pain, so we end up making guesses based on our observations. We used to think that very young children may not experience pain (or remember it) like adults do. We now know that young children do feel pain, and they remember it for a very long time.

Children with chronic pain have significant consequences from it. It's estimated that as many as 40% of these children experience major impacts on appetite, sleep, school performance and attendance, and social engagement and they require multiple medical visits. All of these factors contribute to a decreased quality of life.

A couple of large studies demonstrate that we have treated children's pain differently than adult pain. Eland (1974) completed a small study that contrasted pain dosing for children and adults. The children in this study received 24 analgesic doses for pain compared with 671 doses received by adults with the same conditions. These painful events included amputation of a foot and removal of a kidney.

Swafford and Allan (1968) looked at how many children received medication for pain after general surgery, and the results were astonishing. A mere 3% of children received analgesia after surgery. The assumption appeared to be that the pain experience was somehow different in children than in adults.

While we have a long way to go to have robust research into adults with chronic pain, we are in worse shape in our research on children with chronic pain, even though we know they have it and that it causes untold suffering. We have a solid body of randomized controlled studies exploring adult issues with chronic pain, but far fewer focusing on children. Our treatment of children is often determined by what works for adults, which is a weak foundation on which to base treatment.

A good example of a childhood pain condition for which we have little research is Complex Regional Pain Syndrome. This syndrome often has an onset between the ages of nine and fifteen years, with usual onset between ten and twelve. If we can effectively measure and treat chronic pain in children, we'll see much better outcomes over the course of their lives.

Another area in which we need additional research is in our use of cognitive-behavioral therapy (CBT) with children. CBT techniques are proven to be successful with adults who have chronic pain, but research on children has only been done for chronic headache. There would be an obvious benefit to expanding research into other pain conditions in children.

There are additional factors that distinguish children's chronic pain from that of adults. When children experience pain they tend to react in a more excitable way than adults. It is evident that emotional and social factors such as family dynamics seem to play more of a role in the pain of children. A recent meta-analysis found that the greatest risk factors for pediatric pain are lower socioeconomic status and negative emotional symptoms (Huguet et al., 2016).

> Cognitive approaches can be helpful in building coping skills for these children. CBT can boost children's ability to self-monitor both their emotional and physical states and observe their pain with less judgment and reactivity.

Children experience many of the same responses to chronic pain that adults do—anxiety, depressive symptoms, negative expectations, loss of control, and poor coping skills, all of which contribute to their pain. Other contributors that are similar to those in adults may be withdrawal from activities, frustration, and fear.

While many features of chronic pain are similar in adults and children, there are some things that are more complicated in children. Children may have less understanding of what's going on, they may not utilize alternative therapies as often as adults do (e.g., physical therapy, acupuncture, massage), and parents' emotional upset about the pain may add to their difficulties. Pain in childhood often disrupts school attendance and performance and involvement in sports and extracurricular activities and can negatively impact friendships. Children with chronic pain may be more dependent on their caregivers and for longer and may not fully participate in the work of the family (chores).

Case Example

Sasha – Dealing with a Minor

Sasha is an 11-year-old girl who is brought to your office by her father. He is worried about Sasha's health challenges and how she's handling them. He remarks:

> *"Sasha developed horrible stomach problems after she turned nine. She hurt all the time, felt nauseated almost every day, and even threw up at school a couple of times. Once that happened, she was so embarrassed that she didn't want to go to school at all. We took her to several doctors, and nobody could figure out what's going on. Finally, after two years of this, she got diagnosed with reflux. At least we have an answer, but it actually hasn't fixed her problems. This has messed her up."*

As her father is talking, Sasha is quietly taking it in. As you ask her how this is affecting her, she takes a moment to think, then says:

> *"I haven't been able to eat pizza with my friends. Almost everything I eat upsets my stomach, so I feel weird and different. I had to quit soccer because I was afraid I'd throw up on the field. I've been absent from school a lot, and now I have to go to Saturday school. I can't believe I'm going to feel this bad forever. It scares me. And my parents are always asking me how I am, and I get tired of that. The answer is always the same . . . I feel bad."*

Parental responses to their child being in pain play a big role in the child's progress or lack thereof. When caregivers expect a diagnosis and a "fix" for their child's pain, they may aggressively pursue multiple specialty physician appointments, testing, and other diagnostic aids, and when no clear explanation for the pain is found, they may step up their energetic pursuit of an answer. The challenge of accepting that the pain is chronic, there isn't a clear diagnostic cause, and that emotional factors play a role is often a hard pill for caregivers to swallow. Parents' determination to continue seeking a "reason" for the pain may delay its effective management. Waiting on an "answer" may end up taking a lot of time that could be better spent practicing some helpful coping skills.

An additional issue for these families is the likelihood of caregivers catastrophizing about their child's pain. This increases stress for both the caregivers and the child. What's more, when parents have difficulty accepting and appropriately responding to the child's pain, it increases the risk of disability in the future.

Caregivers are likely to be more accepting of their child's condition if the clinician explains that the pain is chronic but can be treated even in the absence of a clear diagnosis. If we can help parents understand that modifying the emotions and cognitions of the child (as well as their own) can help, then we are much more likely to see improvement.

ETHICAL ISSUES WITH THE ELDERLY

There are a multitude of ethical issues involved with elderly individuals who have chronic pain. For one thing, a lot of older adults (and professionals) figure that pain is a normal part of aging, so they don't vigorously treat it. This is a disservice to older people, who may end up gritting their teeth and putting up with pain, not realizing they can do something to bring relief.

The list of risk factors for pain in the elderly is sobering and includes older age, low socioeconomic status, lower education level, obesity, tobacco use, history of injury, childhood trauma, and coexisting depression and anxiety. Chronic pain in elderly people is associated with reduced activity, falls, mood changes, sleep problem, isolation, and disability.

> Chronic pain in elderly people is associated with reduced activity, falls, mood changes, sleep problems, isolation, and disability.

There are many comorbid conditions that go along with chronic pain in the elderly. Depression, disability, social isolation, and general medical decline all contribute to the challenges that elderly people face. Older people may also have neurocognitive impairments that impact their ability to articulate or accurately report pain. Perhaps someone with dementia lacks the ability to communicate discomfort in a way that can be understood. In these cases, mindfulness approaches may be more effective than cognitive treatment. It's estimated that in long-term care facilities, about 80% of residents have chronic pain. Care facility residents are also the people most likely to have dementia or communication impairments that limit the ability to report their pain accurately. Underreporting pain may be related to a fear of being hospitalized, a desire to please the physician and be seen as compliant, or a generational belief or intrinsic value that pain should be tolerated and not complained about.

Treatment options are more limited in the elderly. All of the medications used for pain pose more risks to and produce more side effects in the elderly. Many of the procedures used for chronic pain may also carry more risk and therefore have limited application in this population. This makes the use of behavioral treatment all the more important.

ETHICAL ISSUES IN MINORITY POPULATIONS

There are clear and disturbing patterns in chronic pain in minority populations. Overall, people of racial and ethnic minorities receive a poorer quality of pain care. It seems that their complaints of pain are taken less seriously than those of majority populations and that their pain is treated less aggressively. There are many co-occurring conditions that are more common in minorities, especially post-traumatic stress disorder, anxiety, and depression, which make chronic pain more intractable. Statistically, people of color are more likely to live in poverty, which also contributes to worse outcomes. Ironically, people of color are less likely to seek counseling to deal with some of these issues.

People of racial and ethnic minorities are less likely to have health insurance to pay for pain treatment and may have less access to care. They make up about half of uninsured U.S. residents. Even when people of color have the same condition, insurance, and income as whites, their outcomes are worse.

People of color report higher pain scores, greater pain severity and duration, more comorbid conditions, more intense suffering, and less control of pain. They are more likely to report sleep problems and higher levels of disability. When people of color experience post-traumatic stress disorder, they report greater symptom severity and more symptoms overall.

Workers' compensation studies present some interesting findings about people of color and chronic pain: They are twice as likely to be disabled six months after a work-related back injury than whites. People of color who don't have an attorney (which can be costly) have worse outcomes overall, partly due to receiving less medical care and attention.

Key Points of Ethics and Pain Treatment

Important ethical considerations in the treatment of pain include:

- **Beneficence:** In all that we do, we should attempt to help people.

- **Non-maleficence:** In all that we do, we should try not to hurt people.

- **Autonomy:** People should be able to choose their care and treatment when they are able to make these decisions.

- **Justice:** Everyone is treated equally.

- Ethical concerns with **children** involve ineffective or minimal treatment of pain, a lack of research into chronic pain in children, and a scarcity of outcomes research on behavioral treatment.

- **Elderly** people often don't report pain accurately, have more pain-causing conditions, and experience more side effects from pain medication.

- Ethical issues with **minority** populations include poorer quality pain treatment related to poverty, lack of health insurance, less aggressive pain treatment, and more comorbid symptoms relative to majority populations.

Chapter 12

A Path for Treatment -
A Session-by-Session Guide

Throughout this book we've talked about pain and its devastating impact on people, including central sensitization and opioid concerns, and there are myriad treatment options. This chapter provides you with an outline for treatment along with resources from the text. You will have a structure for your work and a direction to go with people who come to you in pain.

You may use this guide with individuals or with groups. This approach can be very effective when used in a group format. Including family members in treatment, either group or individual, can be a strong way to intervene by using the family as part of a healing plan.

You may modify this outline to meet your needs. Bear in mind that treatment may go on longer than the ten sessions that we present here. Use your clinical judgment to discern how you might best tailor this to the needs of the individual (or group) that you are working with. You may spend several sessions on one topic area, or you might find that you need less time than this outline indicates. The important thing is to cover most of these areas in a way that is meaningful for your client.

Session 1: Evaluation

In this initial session you will be doing your evaluation of the client. Much of this is drawn from Chapters 2 and 5.

Possible things to include may be:

Pain interview: This is on page 49

Stages of Change discussed on pages 44-45, as well as My Own Readiness to change exercise on page 46

Self-report measures as listed on page 53 and 54

Pain Catastrophizing Scale: This may be found on page 62

Session 2: Education

You may refer to Chapters 1 and 4 for more details on what you might include in this session. This will provide people with solid and accurate information about chronic pain, central sensitization, and the impact of pain.

Possible tools to introduce are:

Chronic pain cycle as shown on page 13

You may also decide to share the information about the behavioral and psychological and behavioral aspects of chronic pain found on pages 15-18

Central Sensitization Inventory, found on page 8 and 9

You can assess the impact of the person's pain by using the worksheet on page 19

Session 3: Goals and Breathing

Setting goals early in the treatment process provides a path forward. Movement and progress may be unfocused and minimal if goals aren't clear. More information about goal-setting is in Chapter 6. Details about breathing are in Chapter 8.

The best tool for this task is:

SMART goals worksheet on page 72

It's likely that you can complete the goal-setting process and move on to a breathing exercise. While this may seem like an unlikely pairing for a session, it allows you to introduce the value of breathing early in the treatment process.

It may be helpful for you to use the following tools related to breathing practice:

Breathing exercise on page 89

Breathing, Practice Log on page 90

Session 4: The Trauma Triangle

Since a history of trauma is so common for people with chronic pain (and opioid use issues) you may choose to talk about trauma and common emotional reactions to being in chronic pain. You can read more about trauma and the emotional aspect of pain in Chapter 3.

Worksheets for this session would be:

ACE (Adverse Childhood Experiences) Study questions on page 26

You may also want to highlight the common emotional reactions to pain (anger, fear, anxiety, depression, pessimism, and learned helplessness) that are found on page 23 and 24

Session 5: Cognitive-Behavioral Tools, Part 1

In this first discussion of CBT approaches you could cover several areas. Background on this is in Chapter 9.

Suggested worksheets are:

ABC worksheet on page 102

Thought distortions described on page 105

Session 6: Cognitive-Behavioral Tools, Part 2

As a follow up to Session 5, you can introduce additional cognitive-behavioral tools to expand the person's awareness of the role thoughts play in the suffering associated with pain.

Additional resources are:

Automatic Negative Thoughts (ANTS!) worksheet on page 109

Downward Arrow: Page 111

Decatastrophizing: Worksheet on page 114

Session 7: Mindful Practices, Part 1

Mindful practices are a significant component of successful pain treatment. They calm reactivity, provide stress relief, and reduce pain. Chapter 8 covers mindfulness in detail.

In this session the following tools from the text will be useful:

Imagery worksheet on page 92

Meditation exercise, which is on page 95

Session 8: Mindful Practices, Part 2

In order to devote sufficient time to introduce mindful approaches to pain we have divided some of these interventions into two sessions.

These tools will be helpful during this session:

The Relaxation Response as described on page 86 and 87

Progressive Muscle Relaxation exercise found on page 97

Session 9: Additional Treatment Components

In this session you can address several aspects of pain treatment. People are able to implement these ideas with relative ease, and, with practice, will incorporate them into their own pain management program. You'll find more details about these treatment options in Chapter 10.

Useful worksheets for this session are:

Pain tracking worksheet on page 118

Pleasant Activity Scheduling worksheet located on page 120

Time-based pacing, based on the worksheet on page 122

Session 10: Putting It All Together

As you wrap up the active phase of treatment there are a couple of additional items to discuss with clients.

Resources include:

Sleep issues page 123 and 124

Increasing activity level: Information is based on what is presented on page 124

References

For your convenience, purchasers can download and print
worksheets and handouts from www.pesi.com/chronicpain

Afilalo, M., Etropolski, M. S., Kuperwasser, B., Kelly, K., Okamoto, A., Van Hove, I., Haeussler, J. (2010). *Efficacy and Safety of Tapentadol Extended Release Compared with Oxycodone Controlled Release for the Management of Moderate to Severe Chronic Pain Related to Osteoarthritis of the Knee: A Randomized, Double-Blind, Placebo- and Active-Controlled Phase III.* Clin Drug Investig, 30(8), 489–505. https://doi.org/1 [pii]\n10.2165/11533440-000000000-00000

American Psychiatric Association (2013). *Diagnostic and statistical manual of mental disorders.* Washington, D. C.: Author.

Balague, F., Mannion, F., Pellisé, F., & Cedraschi, C. (2011). Non-specific low back pain. *The Lancet, 379,* 482–491. Retrieved from: http://www.thelancet.com/pdfs/journals/lancet/PIIS0140-6736(11)60610-7.pdf

Barke, A., Preis, MA., Schmidt-Samoa, C., Baudewig, J., Kröner-Herwig, B., & Dechent, P. (2016). Neural correlates differ in high and low fear-avoidant chronic low back pain patients when imagining back-straining movements. *Journal of Pain, 17*(8), 930–943.

Benedetti, F., et al. (2002). Placebo analgesia. In *Proceedings of the 10th World Congress on Pain (Progress in Pain Research and Management, Vol. 24)* (pp. 315–323), J. Dostrovsky, D. B. Carr, & M. Koltzenburg (Eds). Seattle: IASP Press.

Benyamin, R., Trescot, A. M., Datta, S., Buenaventura, R., Adlaka, R., Sehgal, N., Vallejo, R. (2008). Opioid complications and side effects. *Pain Physician, 11,* 105–120.

Bingel, U., Wanigasekera, V., Weich, K., Ni Mhuircheartaigh, R., Lee, M. C., Ploner, M., & Tracey, I. (2011). The effect of treatment expectations on drug efficacy: Imaging the analgesic benefit of the opioid remifentanil. *Science Translational Medicine, 3*(70), 70ora14.

Caudill, M. (2016). *Managing pain before it manages you.* New York: Guilford Press.

Centers for Disease Control and Prevention, National Center for Health Statistics (2016). Multiple Cause of Death 1999-2015 on CDC WONDER Online Database, released December, 2016. Data are from the Multiple Cause of Death Files, 1999-2015, as compiled from data provided by the 57 vital statistics jurisdictions through the Vital Statistics Cooperative Program. Retrieved from http://wonder.cdc.gov/mcd-icd10.html on May 27, 2017 11:55:26 AM

Cheatle, M. D. (2011). Depression, chronic pain, and suicide by overdose: On the edge. *Pain Medicine (Malden, Mass.), 12*(Suppl 2), S43–S48.

Darnall, B. (2014). *Less pain fewer pills: Avoid the dangers of prescription opioids and gain control over chronic pain.* Boulder, CO: Bull Publishing Company.

De Ruddere, L., Bosmans, M., Crombez, G., & Goubert, L. (2016). Patients are socially excluded when their pain has no medical explanation. *The Journal of Pain, 17*(9), 1028–1035.

Derry, C., Derry, S., & Moore, R. (2013). Single dose oral ibuprofen plus paracetamol (acetaminophen) for acute postoperative pain (Review). Cochrane Database of Systemic Reviews, (6). http://doi.org/10.1002/14651858.CD010210.pub2

Derry, C., Derry, S., Moore, R. A., & McQuay, H. J. (2009). Single dose oral ibuprofen for acute postoperative pain in adults. Cochrane Database of Systematic Reviews (Online), (3), CD001548. http://doi.org/10.1002/14651858.CD001548.pub2

Doidge, N. (2007). *The brain that changes itself.* New York: Penguin Books.

Dowell, D., Haegerich, T., & Chou, R. (2016). CDC guideline for prescribing opioids for chronic pain. *The Journal of American Medicine, 315*(15), 1624–1645.

Ehde, D., Dillworth, T., & Turner, J. (2014). Cognitive-behavioral therapy for individuals with chronic pain: Efficacy, innovations, and directions for research. *American Psychologist, 69*(2), 153–166.

Eland, J. M. (1974). *Children's communication of pain* (Unpublished doctoral dissertation). University of Iowa, Iowa City.

Elvik, R. (2013). Risk of road accident associated with the use of drugs: A systematic review and meta-analysis of evidence from epidemiological studies. *Accident Analysis and Prevention, 60,* 254–267.

Franklin, G. M. (2014). Opioids for chronic noncancer pain: A position paper of the American Academy of Neurology. *Neurology,* 83(14), 1277–84. http://doi.org/10.1212/ WNL.0000000000000839

Gardner, J. (2009). *The mindfulness solution to pain.* Oakland, CA: New Harbinger Publications.

Gaskell, H., Derry, S., Moore, R., & McQuay, H. (2009). Single dose oral oxycodone and oxycodone plus paracetamol (acetaminophen) for acute postoperative pain in adults. Cochrane Database of Systematic Reviews, (3). http://doi.org/10.1002/14651858.CD002763.pub2

Gautam, S., Franzini, L., Mikhail, O. I., Chan, W., & Turner, B. J. (2015). Original longitudinal analysis of opioid analgesic dose and diabetes quality of care measures. *Pain Medicine, 16*(11), 2134–2141.

Goldstein, P., Shamay-Tsoory, S. G., Yellinek, S., & Weissman-Fogel, I. (2016). Empathy predicts an experimental pain reduction during touch. *The Journal of Pain, 17*(10), 1049–1057.

Grosen, K., Drewes, A., Pilegaard, H., Pfeiffer-Jensen, M., Brock, B., & Vase, L. (2016). Situational but not dispositional pain catastrophizing correlates with early postoperative pain in pain-free patients before surgery. *The Journal of Pain, 17*(5), 549–560.

Huguet, A., Tougas, M. E., Hayden, J., McGrath, P. J., Stinson, J. N., & Chambers, C. T. (2016). A systematic review with meta-analysis of childhood and adolescent risk and prognostic factors for musculoskeletal pain. *Pain, 157,* 1. http://doi.org/10.1097/j.pain.0000000000000685

IASP—International Association for the Study of Pain (n.d.). *IASP taxonomy.* Retrieved 2017 from: http://www.iasp-pain.org/Taxonomy#Pain

Incledon, E., O'Connor, M., Giallo, R., Chalkiadis, G. A., & Palmero, T. M. (2016). Child and family antecedents of pain during the transition to adolescence: A longitudinal population-based study. *The Journal of Pain, 17*(11), 1174–1182.

Jackson, T., Tian, P., Wang, Y., Iezzi, T., & Xie, W. (2016). Toward identifying moderators of associations between pre-surgery emotional distress and postoperative pain outcomes: A meta-analysis of longitudinal studies. *The Journal of Pain, 17*(8), 874–888.

Jamison, R. N., Scanlan, E., Matthews, M. L., Jurcik, D. C., & Ross, E. L. (2016). Attitudes of primary care practitioners in managing chronic pain patients prescribed opioids for pain: A prospective longitudinal controlled trial. *Pain Medicine, 17*(1), 99–113. http://doi.org/10.1111/pme.12871

Juch, J. N. S., Maas, E. T., Ostelo, R. W. J. G., Groeneweg, J. G., Kallewaard, J.-W., Koes, B. W., van Tulder, M. W. (2017). Effect of Radiofrequency Denervation on Pain Intensity Among Patients With Chronic Low Back Pain. *JAMA,* 318(1), 14. http://doi.org/10.1001/ jama.2017.7918

Larson, A. M., Ostapowicz, G., Fontana, R. J., Shakil, S. O., & Lee, W. M. (2000). Outcome of acetaminophen-induced: Liver failure in the USA in suicidal vs accidental overdose: Preliminary results of a prospective multi-center trial. In *Hepatology,* Vol. 32(4), pp. 396A–396A). Philadelphia: W. B. Saunders Co.

Lavigne, J. V., Schulein, M. J., & Hahn, Y. S. (1986). Psychological aspects of painful medical conditions in children II: Personality factors, family characteristics and treatment. *Pain, 27*(2), 147–69. Retrieved from: http://www.ncbi.nlm.nih.gov/pubmed/3540811

Levine, J. D., & Gordon, N. C. (1984). Influence of the method of drug administration on analgesic response. *Nature, 312,* 755–756.

Mansour, A. R., Farmer, M. A., Baliki, M. N., & Apkarian, A. V. (2014). Chronic pain: The role of learning and brain plasticity. *Restorative Neurology and Neuroscience, 32*(1), 129–139. http://doi.org/10.3233/RNN-139003

Marchand, S. (2012). *The phenomenon of pain.* Seattle: IASP Press.

Materson, R. S. (1990). Assessment and diagnostic techniques. In R.S. Weiner (Ed.), *Innovations in pain management: A practical guide for clinicians* (pp. 5.1–5.25). Orlando, FL: Paul M. Deutsch & Associates.

McGrath, P. A. (1990). *Pain in children: Nature, assessment, and treatment.* New York: Guilford Press. Retrieved from: http://www.guilford.com/books/Pain-in-Children/ Patricia-McGrath/ 9780898623901

McGrath, P., & Unruh, A. (1987). *Pain in children and adolescents.* Amsterdam: Elsevier. Retrieved from https://books.google.com/books/about/Pain_in_children_and_adolescents.html?id= DeFsAAAAMAAJ

McHugh, R., Weiss, R., Cornelius, M., Martel, M., Jamison, R., & Edwards, R. (2016). Distress intolerance and prescription opioid misuse among patients with chronic pain. *The Journal of Pain, 17*(7), 806–814.

Moore, R. A., Derry, S., McQuay, H. J., & Wiffen, P. J. (2011). Single dose oral analgesics for acute postoperative pain in adults. Cochrane Database of Systematic Reviews (Online), 9(9), CD008659. http://doi.org/10.1002/14651858.CD008659.pub2

Murphy, J., McKellar, J., Raffa, S., Clark, M., Kerns, R., & Karlin, B. (n.d.). *Cognitive behavioral therapy for chronic pain among veterans: Therapist manual.* Washington, D. C.: U. S. Department of Veterans Affairs.

Nahin, R. L., Boineau, R., Khalsa, P. S., Stussman, B. J., & Weber, W. J. (2016). Evidence-Based Evaluation of Complementary Health Approaches for Pain Management in the United States. *Mayo Clinic Proceedings, 91*(9), 1292–1306. http://doi.org/10.1016/j.mayocp.2016.06.007

Nijs, J., Leysen, L., Adriaenssens, N., Aguilar Ferrándiz, M. E., Devoogdt, N., Tassenoy, A., Meeus, M. (2016). Pain following cancer treatment: Guidelines for the clinical classification of predominant neuropathic, nociceptive and central sensitization pain. *Acta Oncologica, 55*(6), 659–663. http://doi.org/10.3109/0284186X.2016.1167958

O'Keeffe, M., Purtill, H., Kennedy, N., Conneely, M., Hurley, J., O'Sullivan, P., Dankaerts, W., O'Sullivan, K. (2016). Comparative effectiveness of conservative interventions for nonspecific chronic spinal pain: Physical, behavioral/psychological informed, or combined? A systematic review and meta-analysis. *The Journal of Pain, 17*(7), 755–774.

Olivieri, P., Solitar, B., & Dubois, M. (2012). Childhood risk factors for developing fibromyalgia. *Open Access Rheumatology: Research and Reviews, 4*, 109. http://doi.org/10.2147/OARRR. S36086

Ostelo, R. W. J. G., Deyo, R. A., Stratford, P., Waddell, G., Croft, P., Korff, M. Von, De Vet, H. C. (2008). Interpreting change scores for pain and functional status in low back pain towards international consensus regarding minimal important change. *Spine, 33*(1), 90–94. http://doi. org/10.1097/BRS.0b013e31815e3a10

Otis, J. (2007). *Managing chronic pain: A cognitive-behavioral therapy approach (Treatments that work).* New York: Oxford University Press.

Pelletier, R., Higgins, J., & Bourbonnais, D. (2015). Is neuroplasticity in the central nervous system the missing link to our understanding of chronic musculoskeletal disorders? *BMC Musculoskeletal Disorders, 16*(1), 25. http://doi.org/10.1186/s12891-015-0480-y

Poonai, N., Bhullar, G., Lin, K., Papini, A., Mainprize, D., Howard, J., Ali, S. (2014). Oral administration of morphine versus ibuprofen to manage postfracture pain in children: A randomized trial. *Canadian Medical Association Journal, 186*(18), 1358–1363. http://doi. org/10.1503/cmaj.140907

Prochaska, J. O., Norcross, J., & DiClemente, C., (2007). *Changing for good: A revolutionary six-stage program for overcoming bad habits and moving your life positively forward.* New York: HarperCollins.

Schatman, M. (2007). *Ethical issues in chronic pain management.* New York: Informa Healthcare.

Shaheed, C. A., Maher, C. G., Williams, K. A., Day, R., & Mclachlan, A. J. (2016). Efficacy, tolerability, and dose-dependent effects of opioid analgesics for low back pain: A systematic review and meta-analysis. *JAMA Internal Medicine, 176*(7), 958–968. http://doi. org/10.1001/ jamainternmed.2016.1251

Siegel, R. (2016). Beyond symptom management: Mindfulness for chronic pain. Retrieved from: http://pcss-o.org/event/beyond-symptom-management-mindfulness-for-chronic- pain/

Songer, D. (2005). Psychotherapeutic approaches in the treatment of pain. *Psychiatry (Edgmont), 2*(5), 19–24.

Sullivan, M. (2009). *The Pain Catastrophizing Scale user manual.* Montreal, Quebec: McGill University.

Swafford, L. I., & Allan, D. (1968). Pain relief in the pediatric patient. *Medical Clinics of North America, 52*, 131–146.

Tarone, R. E., Blot, W. J., & McLaughlin, J. K. (2004). Nonselective nonaspirin nonsteroidal anti-inflammatory drugs and gastrointestinal bleeding: Relative and absolute risk estimates from recent epidemiologic studies. *American Journal of Therapeutics, 11*(1), 17–25.

Teater, D. (2014). *Evidence for the efficacy of pain medications.* Itasca, IL: National Safety Council. Retrieved from: http://www.nsc.org/RxDrugOverdoseDocuments/Evidence-Efficacy-Pain-Medications.pdf.

Teater, D. (2014). *The psychological and physical side effects of pain medications.* Itasca, IL: National Safety Council. Retrieved from: http://safety.nsc.org/sideeffects

Toms, L., Mcquay, H., Derry, S., & Moore, R. (2008). Single dose oral paracetamol (acetaminophen) for postoperative pain in adults. Cochrane Database of Systematic Reviews, (4). http://doi.org/ 10.1002/14651858.CD004602.pub2

Toms, L., McQuay, H. J., Derry, S., & Moore, R. A. (2008). Single dose oral paracetamol (acetaminophen) with codeine for postoperative pain in adults. Cochrane Database of Systematic Reviews (Online), (4), CD004602. http://doi.org/10.1002/14651858. CD004602.pub2

Turk, D., & Winter, F. (2006). *The pain survival guide: How to reclaim your life.* Washington, D. C.: American Psychological Association.

Veliz, P., Epstein-Ngo, Q. M., Meier, E., Ross-Durow, P. L., Boyd, C. J., & McCabe, S. E. (2014). Painfully obvious: A longitudinal examination of medical use and misuse of opioid medication among adolescent sports participants. *Journal of Adolescent Health, 54*(3), 333–340.

Younger, J. W., Chu, L. F., D'Arcy, N. T., Trott, K. E., Jastrzab, L. E., & Mackey, S. C. (2011). Prescription opioid analgesics rapidly change the human brain. *Pain, 152*(8), 1803–1810. http://doi.org/10.1016/j.pain.2011.03.028

Additional Resources

Post-Kaiser survey of long-term prescription opioid painkiller users. (2016). Retrieved April 15, 2017, from https://www.washingtonpost.com/page/2010-2019/WashingtonPost/2016/12/09/National-Politics/Polling/release_455.xml?tid=a_inl

Tauben, D. (n.d.). The Pain Patient Interview. Retrieved April 15, 2017, from: http://chroniccare.rehab.washington.edu/resources/documents/paininterviewformedstudents.pdf

Wong-Baker FACES Foundation (2016). Wong-Baker FACES® Pain Rating Scale. Retrieved with permission from: http://www.WongBakerFACES.org. Originally published in Whaley & Wong's Nursing Care of Infants and Children. © Elsevier Inc.